MW00718811

THE ITALIAN FOOD 2022

AUTHENTIC REGIONAL RECIPES OF THE TRADITION

ENZO PICCOLO

TABLE OF CONTENTS

Grilled Marinated Pork Chops

Braciole di Maiale ai Ferri

Makes 6 servings

This is a great recipe for quick summer dinners. To test pork chops for doneness, make a small cut near the bone. The meat should still be slightly pink.

1 cup dry white wine

$\frac{1}{4}$ cup olive oil

1 small onion, thinly sliced

1 garlic clove, finely chopped

1 tablespoon chopped fresh rosemary

1 tablespoon chopped fresh sage

6 center-cut pork loin chops, about $\frac{3}{4}$ inch thick

Lemon wedges, for garnish

1. Combine the wine, oil, onion, garlic, and herbs in a baking dish large enough to hold the chops in a single layer. Add the chops, cover, and refrigerate for at least 1 hour.

2. Place a barbecue grill or broiler rack about 5 inches from the heat source. Preheat the grill or broiler. Pat the chops dry with paper towels.

3. Grill the meat 5 to 8 minutes, or until nicely browned. Turn the chops over with tongs and cook on the other side for 6 minutes, or until browned and just slightly pink when cut near the bone. Serve hot, garnished with lemon wedges.

Spareribs, Friuli Style

Spuntature di Maiale alla Friulana

Makes 4 to 6 servings

In Fruili, spareribs are simmered slowly until the meat is tender and falling away from the bone. Serve them with mashed potatoes or a plain risotto.

2 cups homemade Meat Broth or store-bought beef broth

3 pounds pork spareribs, cut into individual ribs

¾ cup all-purpose flour

Salt and freshly ground black pepper

3 tablespoons olive oil

1 large onion, chopped

2 medium carrots, chopped

½ cup dry white wine

1. Prepare the broth, if necessary. Pat the ribs dry with paper towels.

2. On a piece of wax paper, combine the flour and salt and pepper to taste. Roll the ribs in the flour, then shake them to remove the excess.

3. In a wide heavy saucepan, heat the oil over medium heat. Add as many ribs as will fit comfortably in a single layer and brown them well on all sides, about 15 minutes. Transfer the ribs to a plate. Repeat until all of the ribs are browned. Drain off all but 2 tablespoons of the fat.

4. Add the onion and carrots to the pan. Cook, stirring occasionally, until lightly browned, about 10 minutes. Add the wine and cook 1 minute, scraping up and blending in the browned bits at the bottom of the pan with a wooden spoon. Return the ribs to the pan and add the broth. Bring the liquid to a simmer. Reduce the heat to low, cover, and cook, stirring occasionally, about $1^1/_2$ hours, or until the meat is very tender and coming away from the bones. (Add water if the meat becomes too dry.)

5. Transfer the ribs to a warm serving platter and serve immediately.

Spareribs with Tomato Sauce

Spuntature al Pomodoro

Makes 4 to 6 servings

My husband and I had spareribs like these at a favorite osteria, a casual family-style restaurant in Rome called Enoteca Corsi. It is only open for lunch, and the menu is very limited. But every day it is packed with hordes of workers from nearby offices attracted by its very fair prices and delicious homestyle food.

2 tablespoons olive oil

3 pounds pork spareribs, cut into individual ribs

Salt and freshly ground black pepper

1 medium onion, finely chopped

1 medium carrot, finely chopped

1 tender celery rib, finely chopped

2 garlic cloves, finely chopped

4 sage leaves, chopped

½ cup dry white wine

2 cups canned crushed tomatoes

1. In a Dutch oven or wide, heavy saucepan, heat the oil over medium heat. Add just enough of the ribs to fit comfortably in the pan. Brown them well on all sides, about 15 minutes. Transfer the ribs to a plate. Sprinkle with salt and pepper. Continue with the remaining ribs. When all are done, spoon off all but 2 tablespoons of the fat.

2. Add the onion, carrot, celery, garlic, and sage, and cook until wilted, about 5 minutes. Stir in the wine and bring to a simmer 1 minute, stirring with a wooden spoon and scraping up and blending in the browned bits at the bottom of the pan.

3. Return the ribs to the pan. Add the tomatoes, and salt and pepper to taste. Cook 1 to 1½ hours, or until the ribs are very tender and the meat is coming away from the bones.

4. Transfer ribs and tomato sauce to a serving plate and serve immediately.

Spiced Ribs, Tuscan Style

Spuntature alla Toscana

Makes 4 to 6 servings

With friends from the Lucini olive oil company, I visited the home of olive growers in the Chianti region of Tuscany. Our group of journalists ate lunch in a grove of olive trees. After various bruschette and salami, we were served steak, sausages, ribs, and vegetables, all grilled over grapevine cuttings. The pork ribs marinated in a tasty rub of olive oil and crushed spices were my favorite, and we all tried to guess what was in the mix. Cinnamon and fennel were easy, but we were all surprised to learn another spice was star anise. I like to use little baby-back ribs for this recipe, but spareribs would be fine, too.

2 star anise

1 tablespoon fennel seeds

6 juniper berries, lightly crushed with the side of a heavy knife

1 tablespoon kosher or fine sea salt

1 teaspoon cinnamon

1 teaspoon finely ground black pepper

Pinch of crushed red pepper

4 tablespoons olive oil

4 pounds baby-back ribs, cut into individual ribs

1. In a spice grinder or blender, combine the star anise, fennel, juniper, and salt. Grind until fine, about 1 minute.

2. In a large shallow bowl, combine the contents of the spice grinder with the cinnamon and black and red pepper. Add the oil and stir well. Rub the mixture all over the ribs. Place the ribs in the bowl. Cover with plastic wrap and refrigerate 24 hours, stirring occasionally.

3. Place a barbecue grill or broiler rack about 6 inches from the heat source. Preheat the grill or broiler. Pat the ribs dry, then grill or broil the ribs, turning them frequently, until browned and cooked through, about 20 minutes. Serve hot.

Spareribs and Beans

Puntini e Fagioli

Makes 6 servings

When I know I have a busy week ahead, I like to make up stews like this one. They only improve when made in advance, and need just a quick reheating to make a satisfying dinner. Serve these with cooked greens like spinach or escarole, or a green salad.

2 tablespoons olive oil

3 pounds country-style pork spareribs, cut into individual ribs

1 onion, chopped

1 carrot, chopped

1 garlic clove, finely chopped

2½ pounds fresh tomatoes, peeled, seeded, and chopped, or 1 (28-ounce) can peeled tomatoes, chopped

1 (3-inch) sprig rosemary

1 cup water

Salt and freshly ground black pepper

3 cups cooked or canned cannellini or cranberry beans, drained

1. In a large Dutch oven or other deep, heavy pot with a tight-fitting lid, heat the oil over medium heat. Add just enough of the ribs to fit comfortably in the pan. Brown them well on all sides, about 15 minutes. Transfer the ribs to a plate. Sprinkle with salt and pepper. Continue with the remaining ribs. When all are done, pour off all but 2 tablespoons of the fat.

2. Add the onion, carrot, and garlic to the pot. Cook, stirring frequently, until the vegetables are tender, about 10 minutes. Add the ribs, then the tomatoes, rosemary, water, and salt and pepper to taste. Bring to a simmer over low heat and cook 1 hour.

3. Add the beans, cover, and cook 30 minutes or until the meat is very tender and coming away from the bone. Taste and adjust seasoning. Serve hot.

Spicy Pork Chops with Pickled Peppers

Braciole di Maiale con Peperoncini

Makes 4 servings

Pickled hot chiles and sweet pickled peppers are a fine topping for juicy pork chops. Adjust the proportions of the chiles and sweet peppers to suit your taste. Serve these with fried potatoes.

2 tablespoons olive oil

4 center-cut pork loin chops, each about 1 inch thick

Salt and freshly ground black pepper

4 garlic cloves, thinly sliced

1½ cups sliced pickled sweet peppers

¼ cup sliced pickled hot peppers, such as peperoncini or jalapeños, or more of the sweet peppers

2 tablespoons pickling juice or white wine vinegar

2 tablespoons chopped fresh flat-leaf parsley

1. In a large heavy skillet, heat the oil over medium-high heat. Pat the chops dry with paper towels then sprinkle them with salt and pepper. Cook the chops until browned, about 2 minutes, then turn them over with tongs and brown on the other side, about 2 minutes more.

2. Reduce the heat to medium. Scatter the garlic slices around the chops. Cover the pan and cook 5 to 8 minutes or until the chops are tender and just slightly pink when cut near the bone. Regulate the heat so that the garlic does not become dark brown. Transfer the chops to a serving platter and cover to keep warm.

3. Add the sweet and hot peppers and pickling juice or vinegar to the skillet. Cook, stirring, for 2 minutes or until the peppers are heated through and the juices are syrupy.

4. Stir in the parsley. Spoon the contents of the pan over the chops and serve immediately.

Pork Chops with Rosemary and Apples

Braciole al Mele

Makes 4 servings

The sweet-tart flavor of apples is a perfect complement to pork chops. This recipe is from Friuli– Venezia Giulia.

4 center-cut pork chops, each about 1 inch thick

Salt and freshly ground black pepper

1 tablespoon chopped fresh rosemary

1 tablespoon unsalted butter

4 golden delicious apples, peeled and cut into $\frac{1}{2}$-inch pieces

$\frac{1}{2}$ cup Chicken Broth

1. Pat the meat dry with paper towels. Sprinkle the chops on both sides with the salt, pepper, and rosemary.

2. In a large heavy skillet, melt the butter over medium heat. Add the chops and cook until they are nicely browned on one side, about 2 minutes. Turn the chops over with tongs and brown on the other side, about 2 minutes more.

3. Scatter the apples around the chops and pour in the broth. Cover the skillet and turn the heat to low. Cook about 5 to 10 minutes, turning the chops once, until they are tender and just slightly pink when cut near the bone. Serve immediately.

Pork Chops with Mushroom-Tomato Sauce

Costolette di Maiale con Funghi

Makes 4 servings

When buying pork chops, look for chops of similar size and thickness so that they will cook evenly. White button mushrooms, wine, and tomatoes are the sauce for these pork chops. This same treatment is also good on veal chops.

4 tablespoons olive oil

4 center-cut pork loin chops, each about 1 inch thick

Salt and freshly ground black pepper

½ cup dry white wine

1 cup chopped fresh or canned tomatoes

1 tablespoon chopped fresh rosemary

1 (12-ounce) package white mushrooms, lightly rinsed, stemmed, and halved or quartered if large

1. In a large heavy skillet, heat 2 tablespoons of the oil over medium heat. Sprinkle the chops with salt and pepper. Place the chops in the pan in a single layer. Cook until they are nicely browned on one side, about 2 minutes. Turn the chops over with tongs and brown on the other side, about 1 to 2 minutes more. Transfer the chops to a plate.

2. Add the wine to the skillet and bring to a simmer. Add the tomatoes, rosemary, and salt and pepper to taste. Cover and cook 10 minutes.

3. Meanwhile, in a medium skillet, heat the remaining 2 tablespoons of oil over medium heat. Add the mushrooms, and salt and pepper to taste. Cook, stirring frequently, until the liquid evaporates and the mushrooms are browned, about 10 minutes.

4. Return the pork chops to the skillet with the tomato sauce. Stir in the mushrooms. Cover and cook 5 to 10 minutes more or until the pork is just cooked through and the sauce is slightly thickened. Serve immediately.

Pork Chops with Porcini and Red Wine

Costolette con Funghi e Vino

Makes 4 servings

Browning chops or other cuts of meat adds flavor and improves their appearance. Always pat the chops dry just before browning them, as surface moisture will cause the meat to steam and not brown. After browning, these chops are simmered with dried porcini and red wine. A touch of heavy cream gives the sauce a smooth texture and rich flavor.

1 ounce dried porcini mushrooms

1½ cups warm water

2 tablespoons olive oil

4 center-cut pork loin chops, about 1 inch thick

Salt and freshly ground black pepper

½ cup dry red wine

¼ cup heavy cream

1. Place the mushrooms in a bowl with the water. Let stand 30 minutes. Lift the mushrooms out of the liquid and rinse them well under running water, paying special attention to the base of the stems where soil collects. Drain, then chop fine. Pour the soaking liquid through a paper coffee filter–lined strainer into a bowl.

2. In a large skillet, heat the oil over medium heat. Pat the chops dry. Place the chops in the pan in a single layer. Cook until they are nicely browned, about 2 minutes. Turn the chops over with tongs and brown on the other side, about 1 to 2 minutes more. Sprinkle with salt and pepper. Transfer the chops to a plate.

3. Add the wine to the skillet and simmer 1 minute. Add the porcini and their soaking liquid. Reduce the heat to low. Simmer 5 to 10 minutes, or until the liquid is reduced. Stir in the cream and cook 5 minutes more.

4. Return the chops to the pan. Cook 5 minutes more, or until the chops are just cooked through and the sauce is thickened. Serve immediately.

Pork Chops with Cabbage

Costolette di Maiale con Cavolo Rosso

Makes 4 servings

Balsamic vinegar adds color and sweetness to red cabbage and offers a nice balance to the pork. It is not necessary to use an aged balsamic vinegar for this recipe. Save it to use as a condiment for cheese or cooked meat.

2 tablespoons olive oil

4 center-cut pork loin chops, about 1 inch thick

Salt and freshly ground black pepper

1 large onion, chopped

2 large garlic cloves, finely chopped

2 pounds red cabbage, cut into thin strips

$\frac{1}{4}$ cup balsamic vinegar

2 tablespoons water

1. In a large skillet, heat the oil over medium heat. Pat the chops dry with paper towels. Add the chops to the pan. Cook until nicely browned, about 2 minutes. Turn the meat over with tongs and brown on the other side, about 1 to 2 minutes more. Sprinkle with salt and pepper. Transfer the chops to a plate.

2. Add the onion to the skillet and cook 5 minutes. Stir in the garlic and cook 1 minute more.

3. Add the cabbage, balsamic vinegar, water, and salt to taste. Cover and cook, stirring occasionally, until the cabbage is tender, about 45 minutes.

4. Add the chops to the pan and cook, turning the chops once or twice in the sauce, until the meat is just cooked through and slightly pink when cut near the bone, about 5 minutes more. Serve immediately.

Pork Chops with Fennel and White Wine

Braciole di Maiale al Vino

Makes 4 servings

There is not a lot of sauce left in the pan when these chops are done, just a tablespoon or two of concentrated glaze to moisten the meat. If you prefer not to use fennel seeds, try substituting a tablespoon of fresh rosemary.

2 tablespoons olive oil

4 center-cut pork loin chops, about 1 inch thick

1 garlic clove, lightly crushed

Salt and freshly ground black pepper

2 teaspoons fennel seeds

1 cup dry white wine

1. In a large skillet, heat the oil over medium-high heat. Pat the pork chops dry. Add the pork chops and garlic to the pan. Cook until the chops are browned, about 2 minutes. Sprinkle with the fennel seeds and the salt and pepper. Turn the chops over with tongs and brown on the second side, about 1 to 2 minutes more.

2. Add the wine and bring to a simmer. Cover and cook 3 to 5 minutes or until the chops are cooked through and just pink when cut near the bone.

3. Transfer the chops to a plate and discard the garlic. Cook the pan juices until reduced and syrupy. Pour the juices over the chops and serve immediately.

Pork Chops, Pizzamaker's Style

Braciole alla Pizzaiola

Makes 4 servings

In Naples, pork chops and small steaks, too, can be prepared alla pizzaiola, in the style of the pizzamaker. The sauce is typically served over spaghetti as a first course. The chops are served as a second course with a green salad. There should be just enough sauce for a half-pound of spaghetti, with a spoonful or so left to serve with the chops.

2 tablespoons olive oil

4 pork rib chops, about 1 inch thick

Salt and freshly ground black pepper

2 large garlic cloves, finely chopped

1 (28-ounce) can peeled tomatoes, drained and chopped

1 teaspoon dried oregano

Pinch crushed red pepper

2 tablespoons chopped fresh flat-leaf parsley

1. In a large skillet, heat the oil over medium heat. Pat the chops dry and sprinkle with salt and pepper. Add the chops to the pan. Cook until the chops are browned, about 2 minutes. Turn the chops over with tongs and brown on the other side, about 2 minutes more. Transfer the chops to a plate.

2. Add the garlic to the pan and cook 1 minute. Add the tomatoes, oregano, red pepper, and salt to taste. Bring the sauce to a simmer. Cook, stirring occasionally, 20 minutes or until the sauce is thickened.

3. Return the chops to the sauce. Cook 5 minutes, turning the chops once or twice, until they are just cooked through and slightly pink when cut near the bone. Sprinkle with parsley. Serve immediately, or if using the sauce for spaghetti, cover the chops with foil to keep warm.

Pork Chops, Molise Style

Pampanella Sammartinese

Makes 4 servings

These chops are spicy and unusual. At one time cooks in Molise would dry their own sweet red peppers in the sun to make paprika. Today, commercially made sweet paprika is used in Italy. In the United States, use paprika imported from Hungary for best flavor.

Grilling pork chops is tricky because they can dry out so easily. Watch them carefully and cook them only until the meat is just slightly pink near the bone.

¼ cup sweet paprika

2 garlic cloves, chopped

1 teaspoon salt

Crushed red pepper

2 tablespoons white wine vinegar

4 center-cut pork loin chops, about 1 inch thick

1. In a small bowl, mix together the paprika, garlic, salt, and a generous pinch of crushed red pepper. Add the vinegar and stir until smooth. Place the chops on a plate and brush them on all sides with the paste. Cover and refrigerate 1 hour up to overnight.

2. Place a barbecue grill or broiler rack about 6 inches from the heat source. Preheat the grill or broiler. Cook pork chops until browned on one side, about 6 minutes, then turn the meat over with tongs and brown the other side, about 5 minutes more. Cut into the chops near the bone; the meat should be slightly pink. Serve immediately.

Balsamic-Glazed Pork Tenderloin with Arugula and Parmigiano

Maiale al Balsamico con Insalata

Makes 6 servings

Pork tenderloins are quick-cooking and low in fat. Here, the glazed pork slices are paired with a crisp arugula salad. If you cannot find arugula, substitute watercress.

2 pork tenderloins (about 1 pound each)

1 garlic clove, finely chopped

1 tablespoon balsamic vinegar

1 teaspoon honey

Salt and freshly ground black pepper

Salad

2 tablespoons olive oil

1 tablespoon balsamic vinegar

Salt and freshly ground black pepper

6 cups trimmed arugula, rinsed and dried

A piece of Parmigiano-Reggiano

1. Place a rack in the center of the oven. Preheat the oven to 450°F. Oil a baking pan just large enough to hold the pork.

2. Pat the pork dry with paper towels. Fold the thin ends under to make it an even thickness. Place the tenderloins about an inch apart in the pan.

3. In a small bowl, stir together the garlic, vinegar, honey, and salt and pepper to taste.

4. Brush the mixture over the meat. Place the pork in the oven and roast 15 minutes. Pour $^1/_2$ cup of water around the meat. Roast 10 to 20 minutes more or until browned and tender. (Pork is done when the internal temperature reaches 150°F on an instant-read thermometer.) Remove the pork from the oven. Leave it in the pan and let it rest at least 10 minutes.

5. In a large bowl, whisk together the oil, vinegar, and salt and pepper to taste. Add the arugula and toss with the dressing. Pile the arugula in the center of a large platter or individual dinner plates.

6. Thinly slice the pork and arrange it around the greens. Drizzle with the pan juices. With a swivel-blade vegetable peeler, shave thin slices of Parmigiano-Reggiano over the arugula. Serve immediately.

Herbed Pork Tenderloin

Filetto di Maiale alle Erbe

Makes 6 servings

Pork tenderloins are now readily available, usually packed two to a package. They are lean and tender, if not overcooked, though the flavor is very mild. Grilling gives them added flavor, and they can be served hot or at room temperature.

2 pork tenderloins (about 1 pound each)

2 tablespoons olive oil

2 tablespoons chopped fresh sage

2 tablespoons chopped fresh basil

2 tablespoons chopped fresh rosemary

1 garlic clove, finely chopped

Salt and freshly ground black pepper

1. Pat the meat dry with paper towels. Place the pork tenderloins on a plate.

2. In a small bowl, mix together the oil, herbs, garlic, and salt and pepper to taste. Rub the mixture over the tenderloins. Cover and refrigerate at least 1 hour or up to overnight.

3. Preheat the grill or broiler. Grill the tenderloins 7 to 10 minutes, or until browned. Turn the meat over with tongs and cook 7 minutes more, or until an instant-read thermometer inserted in the center reads 150°F. Sprinkle with salt. Let the meat rest 10 minutes before slicing. Serve hot or at room temperature.

Calabrian-Style Pork Tenderloin with Honey and Chile

Carne 'ncantarata

Makes 6 servings

More than any other region in Italy, cooks in Calabria incorporate chile peppers into their cooking. Chiles are used fresh, dried, ground, or crushed into flakes or powder—as paprika or cayenne.

In Castrovillari, my husband and I ate at the Locanda di Alia, an elegant country restaurant and inn. The region's most famous restaurant is run by the Alia brothers. Gaetano is the chef, while Pinuccio manages the front of the house. Their specialty is pork marinated with fennel and chiles in a honey and chile sauce. Pinuccio explained that the recipe, which is at least two hundered years old, was made with preserved pork that had been salted and cured for several months. This is a more streamlined way of making it.

Fennel pollen can be found at many shops specializing in herbs and spices. (See Sources.) Crushed fennel seeds can be used if the pollen is not available.

2 pork tenderloins (about 1 pound each)

2 tablespoons honey

1 teaspoon salt

1 teaspoon fennel pollen or crushed fennel seeds

Pinch of crushed red pepper

½ cup orange juice

2 tablespoons paprika

1. Place a rack in the center of the oven. Preheat the oven to 425°F. Oil a baking pan just large enough to hold the pork.

2. Fold the thin ends of the tenderloins under to make an even thickness. Place the tenderloins about an inch apart in the pan.

3. In a small bowl, stir together the honey, salt, fennel pollen, and crushed red pepper. Brush the mixture over the meat. Place the pork in the oven and roast 15 minutes.

4. Pour the orange juice around the meat. Roast 10 to 20 minutes more, or until browned and tender. (Pork is done when the internal temperature reaches 150°F on an instant-read thermometer.) Transfer the pork to a cutting board. Cover with foil and keep warm while preparing the sauce.

5. Place the baking pan over medium heat. Stir in the paprika and cook, scraping the bottom of the pan, for 2 minutes.

6. Slice the pork and serve it with the sauce.

Roast Pork with Potatoes and Rosemary

Arista di Maiale con Patate

Makes 6 to 8 servings

Everybody loves this pork roast—it's easy to make, and the potatoes absorb the flavors of the pork as they cook together in the same pan. Irresistible.

1 center-cut boneless pork loin roast (about 3 pounds)

2 tablespoons chopped fresh rosemary

2 tablespoons chopped fresh garlic

4 tablespoons olive oil

Salt and freshly ground black pepper

2 pounds new potatoes, halved, or quartered if large

1. Place a rack in the center of the oven. Preheat the oven to 425°F. Oil a roasting pan large enough to hold the pork and potatoes without crowding.

2. In a small bowl, make a paste with the rosemary, garlic, 2 tablespoons of the oil, and a generous amount of salt and pepper. Toss the potatoes in the pan with the remaining 2 tablespoons of oil and half of the garlic paste. Push the potatoes aside and place the meat fat-side up in the center of the pan. Rub or spread the remaining paste all over the meat.

3. Roast 20 minutes. Turn the potatoes. Reduce the heat to 350°F. Roast 1 hour more, turning the potatoes every 20 minutes. The meat is done when the internal temperature of the pork reaches 150°F on an instant-read thermometer.

4. Transfer the meat to a cutting board. Cover loosely with foil and let rest 10 minutes. The potatoes should be browned and tender. If necessary, turn up the heat and cook them a little more.

5. Slice the meat and arrange it on a warm serving platter surrounded by the potatoes. Serve hot.

Pork Loin with Lemon

Maiale con Limone

Makes 6 to 8 servings

Pork loin roasted with lemon zest makes a fine Sunday dinner. I serve it with slow-cooked cannellini beans and a green vegetable like broccoli or brussels sprouts.

Butterflying the loin is easy enough to do yourself if you follow the instructions; otherwise have the butcher handle it.

1 center-cut boneless pork loin roast (about 3 pounds)

1 teaspoon grated lemon zest

2 garlic cloves, finely chopped

2 tablespoons chopped fresh flat-leaf parsley

2 tablespoons olive oil

Salt and freshly ground black pepper

$\frac{1}{2}$ cup dry white wine

1. Place a rack in the center of the oven. Preheat the oven to 425°F. Oil a roasting pan just large enough to hold the meat.

2. In a small bowl, mix together the lemon zest, garlic, parsley, oil, and salt and pepper to taste.

3. Pat the meat dry with paper towels. To butterfly the pork, place it on a cutting board. With a long sharp knife such as a boning knife or chef's knife, cut the pork almost in half lengthwise, stopping about $3/4$ inch from one long side. Open the meat like a book. Spread the lemon and garlic mixture over the side of the meat. Roll up the pork from one long side to the other like a sausage and tie it with kitchen string at 2-inch intervals. Sprinkle the outside with salt and pepper.

4. Place the meat fat-side up in the prepared pan. Roast 20 minutes. Reduce the heat to 350°F. Roast 40 minutes more. Add the wine and roast 15 to 30 minutes longer, or until the temperature on an instant-read thermometer reaches 150°F.

5. Transfer the roast to a cutting board. Cover the meat loosely with foil. Let rest 10 minutes before slicing. Place the pan on the stove over medium heat and reduce the pan juices slightly. Slice the pork and transfer it to a serving platter. Pour the juices over the meat. Serve hot.

Pork Loin with Apples and Grappa

Maiale con Mele

Makes 6 to 8 servings

Apples and onions teamed with grappa and rosemary flavor this tasty roast pork loin from Friuli–Venezia Giulia.

1 center-cut boneless pork loin roast (about 3 pounds)

1 tablespoon chopped fresh rosemary, plus more for garnish

Salt and freshly ground black pepper

2 tablespoons olive oil

2 Granny Smith or other tart apples, peeled and thinly sliced

1 small onion, thinly sliced

¼ cup grappa or brandy

½ cup dry white wine

1. Place a rack in the center of the oven. Preheat the oven to 350°F. Lightly oil a roasting pan large enough to hold the meat.

2. Rub the pork with the rosemary, salt and pepper to taste, and olive oil. Place the meat fat-side up in the pan and surround it with the apple and onion slices.

3. Pour the grappa and wine over the meat. Roast for 1 hour and 15 minutes, or until an instant-read thermometer inserted in the center reads 150°F. Transfer the meat to a cutting board and cover with foil to keep warm.

4. The apples and onions should be soft. If not, return the pan to the oven and roast 15 minutes more.

5. When they are tender, scrape the apples and onions into a food processor or blender. Puree until smooth. (Add a tablespoon or two of warm water to thin the mixture if needed.)

6. Slice the meat and arrange it on a heated platter. Spoon the apple-onion puree to one side. Garnish with fresh rosemary. Serve hot.

Roast Pork with Hazelnuts and Cream

Arrosto di Maiale alle Nocciole

Makes 6 to 8 servings

This is a variation on a Piedmontese roast pork recipe that first appeared in my book Italian Holiday Cooking. Here cream, along with hazelnuts, enriches the sauce.

1 center-cut boneless pork loin roast (about 3 pounds)

2 tablespoons chopped fresh rosemary

2 large garlic cloves, finely chopped

2 tablespoons olive oil

Salt and freshly ground black pepper

1 cup dry white wine

$\frac{1}{2}$ cup hazelnuts, toasted, skinned, and coarsely chopped (see How To Toast and Skin Nuts)

1 cup homemade Meat Broth or Chicken Broth, or store-bought beef or chicken broth

$\frac{1}{2}$ cup heavy cream

1. Place a rack in the center of the oven. Preheat the oven to 425°F. Oil a roasting pan just large enough to hold the meat.

2. In a small bowl, mix together the rosemary, garlic, oil, and salt and pepper to taste. Place the meat fat-side up in the pan. Rub the garlic mixture all over the pork. Roast the meat 15 minutes.

3. Pour the wine over the meat. Cook 45 to 60 minutes more, or until the temperature of the pork reaches 150°F on an instant-read thermometer and the meat is tender when pierced with a fork. Meanwhile, prepare the hazelnuts, if necessary.

4. Transfer the meat to a cutting board. Cover with foil to keep warm.

5. Place the pan over medium heat on the top of the stove and bring the juices to a simmer. Add the broth and simmer 5 minutes, scraping up and blending in the browned bits on the bottom of the pan with a wooden spoon. Add the cream and simmer until slightly thickened, about 2 minutes more. Stir in the chopped nuts and remove from the heat.

6. Slice the meat and arrange the slices on a warm serving platter. Spoon the sauce over the pork and serve hot.

Tuscan Pork Loin

Arista di Maiale

Makes 6 to 8 servings

Here is a classic Tuscan-style pork roast. Cooking the meat with the bone makes it much more flavorful, and the bones are also great to gnaw on.

3 large garlic cloves

2 tablespoons fresh rosemary

Salt and freshly ground black pepper

2 tablespoons olive oil

1 bone-in center-cut rib roast, about 4 pounds

1 cup dry white wine

1. Place a rack in the center of the oven. Preheat the oven to 325°F. Oil a roasting pan just large enough to hold the roast.

2. Very finely chop the garlic and rosemary together, then place them in a small bowl. Add the salt and pepper to taste and mix well to form a paste. Place the roast fat-side up in the pan. With a

small knife, make deep slits all over the surface of the pork, then insert the mixture into the slits. Rub the roast all over with the olive oil.

3. Roast 1 hour 15 minutes or until the meat reaches an internal temperature of 150°F on an instant-read thermometer. Transfer the meat to a cutting board. Cover with foil to keep warm. Let rest 10 minutes.

4. Place the pan over low heat on the top of the stove. Add the wine and cook, scraping up and blending in the browned bits at the bottom of the pan with a wooden spoon until slightly reduced, about 2 minutes. Pour the juices through a strainer into a bowl and skim off the fat. Reheat if necessary.

5. Slice the meat and arrange it on a warm serving platter. Serve it hot with the pan juices.

Roast Pork Shoulder with Fennel

Porchetta

Makes 12 servings

This is my version of the fabulous roast pig known as porchetta, sold all around central Italy, including Lazio, Umbria, and Abruzzo. Slices of the pork are sold from special trucks, and you can order it on a sandwich or wrapped in paper to take home. Though the meat is luscious, the crackling pork skin is the best part.

The roast is cooked for a long time and to a high temperature because it is very dense. The high fat content keeps the meat moist, and the skin gets brown and crunchy. A fresh ham can be substituted for the pork shoulder.

1 (7-pound) pork shoulder roast

8 to 12 garlic cloves

2 tablespoons chopped fresh rosemary

1 tablespoon fennel seeds

1 tablespoon salt

1 teaspoon freshly ground black pepper

¼ cup olive oil

1. About 1 hour before you begin roasting the meat, remove it from the refrigerator.

2. Very finely chop together the garlic, rosemary, fennel, and salt, then place the seasonings in a small bowl. Stir in the pepper and oil to form a smooth paste.

3. With a small knife, cut deep slits into the surface of the pork. Insert the paste into the slits.

4. Place a rack in the lower third of the oven. Preheat the oven to 350°F. When ready, place the roast in the oven and cook 3 hours. Spoon off the excess fat. Roast the meat 1 to $1^1/_2$ hours longer, or until the temperature reaches 160°F on an instant-read thermometer. When the meat is done, the fat will be crisp and a deep nutty brown.

5. Transfer the meat to a cutting board. Cover with foil to keep warm and let stand 20 minutes. Carve and serve hot or at room temperature.

Roast Suckling Pig

Maialino Arrosto

Makes 8 to 10 servings

A suckling pig is one that has not been allowed to eat adult pig food. In the United States, suckling pigs typically weigh between 15 and 20 pounds, though in Italy they are half that size. Even at the higher weight, there really is not much meat on a suckling pig, so don't plan to serve more than eight to ten guests. Also, be sure you have a very large baking pan to accommodate a whole piglet, which will be about 30 inches long, and be sure your oven will accommodate the pan. Any good butcher should be able to obtain a fresh piglet for you, but make inquiries before planning on it.

Sardinian cooks are famous for their suckling pig, but I have eaten it in many places in Italy. The one I remember best was part of a memorable luncheon enjoyed at the Majo di Norante winery in Abruzzo.

1 suckling pig, about 15 pounds

4 garlic cloves

2 tablespoons chopped fresh flat-leaf parsley

1 tablespoon chopped fresh rosemary

1 tablespoon chopped fresh sage

1 teaspoon juniper berries, chopped

Salt and freshly ground black pepper

6 tablespoons olive oil

2 bay leaves

1 cup dry white wine

Apple, orange, or other fruit for garnish (optional)

1. Place a rack in the lower third of the oven. Preheat the oven to 425°F. Oil a baking pan large enough to hold the pig.

2. Rinse the pig well inside and out and pat dry with paper towels.

3. Chop together the garlic, parsley, rosemary, sage, and juniper berries, then place the seasonings in a small bowl. Add a generous amount of salt and freshly ground pepper. Stir in two tablespoons of the oil.

4. Place the pig on its side on a large roasting rack in the prepared pan and spread the herb mixture inside the body cavity. Add the

bay leaves. Cut slashes about $1/2$ inch deep along both sides of the backbone. Rub the remaining oil all over the surface of the pig. Cover the ears and tail with aluminum foil. (If you want to serve the pig whole with an apple or other fruit in its mouth, prop the mouth open with a ball of aluminum foil about the size of the fruit.) Sprinkle the outside with salt and pepper.

5. Roast the pig 30 minutes. Reduce the heat to 350°F. Baste with the wine. Roast 2 to $2^1/_2$ hours more, or until an instant-read thermometer inserted in the meaty part of the hindquarter registers 170°F. Baste every 20 minutes with the pan juices.

6. Transfer the pig to a large cutting board. Cover with foil and let rest 30 minutes. Remove the foil covering and the ball of foil from the mouth, if using. Replace the foil ball with the fruit, if using. Transfer to a serving platter and serve hot.

7. Skim the fat from the pan juices and reheat them over low heat. Pour the juices over the meat. Serve immediately.

Boneless Spiced Pork Loin Roast

Maiale in Porchetta

Makes 6 to 8 servings

Boneless pork loin is roasted with the same spices used for porchetta (baby pig roasted on a spit) in many parts of central Italy. After a brief period of cooking at high heat, the oven temperature is turned down low, which keeps the meat tender and juicy.

4 garlic cloves

1 tablespoon fresh rosemary

6 fresh sage leaves

6 juniper berries

1 teaspoon salt

$\frac{1}{2}$ teaspoon freshly ground black pepper

1 boneless center-cut pork loin roast, about 3 pounds

Extra-virgin olive oil

1 cup dry white wine

1. Place a rack in the center of the oven. Preheat the oven to 450°F. Oil a roasting pan just large enough to hold the pork.

2. Very finely chop together the garlic, rosemary, sage, and juniper berries. Stir together the herb mixture, the salt, and the pepper.

3. With a large, sharp knife, cut the meat lengthwise down the center, leaving it attached on one side. Open the meat like a book and spread two-thirds of the spice mixture over the meat. Close the meat and tie it with string at 2-inch intervals. Rub the remaining spice mixture over the outside. Place the meat in the pan. Drizzle with olive oil.

4. Roast the pork 10 minutes. Reduce the heat to 300°F and roast 60 minutes more, or until the internal temperature of the pork reaches 150°F.

5. Remove the roast to a serving platter and cover with foil. Let rest 10 minutes.

6. Add the wine to the pan and place it over medium heat on the top of the stove. Cook, scraping up any brown bits in the pan with a wooden spoon, until the juices are reduced and syrupy. Slice the pork and spoon on the pan juices. Serve hot.

Braised Pork Shoulder in Milk

Maiale al Latte

Makes 6 to 8 servings

In Lombardy and the Veneto, veal, pork, and chicken are sometimes cooked in milk. This keeps the meat tender, and when it is done the milk makes a creamy brown sauce to serve with the meat.

Vegetables, pancetta, and wine add flavor. I use a boneless shoulder or butt roast for this dish because it takes well to slow, moist cooking. The meat is cooked on the stove, so you don't need to turn on your oven.

1 boneless pork shoulder or butt roast (about 3 pounds)

4 ounces finely diced pancetta

1 carrot, finely chopped

1 small tender celery rib

1 medium onion, finely chopped

1 quart milk

Salt and freshly ground black pepper

½ cup dry white wine

1. In a large Dutch oven or other deep, heavy pot with a tight-fitting lid, combine the pork, pancetta, carrot, celery, onion, milk, and salt and pepper to taste. Bring the liquid to a simmer over medium heat.

2. Partially cover the pot and cook over medium heat, turning occasionally, about 2 hours or until the meat is tender when pierced with a fork.

3. Transfer the meat to a cutting board. Cover with foil to keep warm. Raise the heat under the pot and cook until the liquid is reduced and lightly browned. Pour the juices through a strainer into a bowl, then pour the liquid back into the pot

4. Pour the wine into the pot and bring to a simmer, scraping up and blending in any browned bits with a wooden spoon. Slice the pork and arrange it on a warm serving platter. Pour the cooking liquid over the top. Serve hot.

Braised Pork Shoulder with Grapes

Maiale all' Uva

Makes 6 to 8 servings

Pork shoulder or butt is particularly good for braising. It stays nice and moist despite the long simmering. I used to make this Sicilian recipe with pork loin, but I now find that the loin is too lean and shoulder has more flavor.

1 pound pearl onions

3 pounds boneless pork shoulder or butt, rolled and tied

2 tablespoons olive oil

Salt and freshly ground black pepper

¼ cup white wine vinegar

1 pound seedless green grapes, stemmed (about 3 cups)

1. Bring a large pot of water to a boil. Add the onions and cook for 30 seconds. Drain and cool under cold running water.

2. With a sharp paring knife, shave off the tip of the root ends. Do not slice off the ends too deeply or the onions will fall apart during cooking. Remove the skins.

3. In a Dutch oven just large enough to hold the meat or another deep, heavy pot with a tight-fitting lid, heat the oil over medium-high heat. Pat the pork dry with paper towels. Place the pork in the pot and brown well on all sides, about 20 minutes. Tip the pot and spoon off the fat. Sprinkle the pork with salt and pepper.

4. Add the vinegar and bring it to a simmer, scraping up the browned bits at the bottom of the pot with a wooden spoon. Add the onions and 1 cup water. Reduce the heat to low and simmer 1 hour.

5. Add the grapes. Cook 30 minutes more or until the meat is very tender when pierced with a fork. Transfer the meat to a cutting board. Cover with foil to keep warm and let sit 15 minutes.

6. Slice the pork and arrange it on a warm serving platter. Spoon on the grape and onion sauce and serve immediately.

Beer-Braised Pork Shoulder

Maiale alla Birra

Makes 8 servings

Fresh pork shanks are cooked this way in Trentino– Alto Adige, but since that cut is not widely available in the United States, I use the same flavorings to cook a bone-in shoulder roast. There will be a lot of fat at the end of the cooking time, but this can easily be skimmed off the surface of the cooking liquid. Better yet, cook the pork a day ahead of serving and chill the meat and cooking juices separately. The fat will harden and can easily be removed. Reheat the pork in the cooking liquid before serving.

5 to 7 pounds bone-in pork shoulder (picnic or Boston butt)

Salt and freshly ground black pepper

2 tablespoons olive oil

1 medium onion, finely chopped

2 garlic cloves, finely chopped

2 sprigs fresh rosemary

2 bay leaves

12 ounces beer

1. Pat the pork dry with paper towels. Sprinkle the meat all over with salt and pepper.

2. In a large Dutch oven or other deep, heavy pot with a tight-fitting lid, heat the oil over medium heat. Place the pork in the pot and brown it well on all sides, about 20 minutes Spoon off all but 1 or 2 tablespoons of the fat.

3. Scatter the onion, garlic, rosemary, and bay leaves all around the meat and cook 5 minutes. Add the beer and bring to a simmer.

4. Cover the pot and cook, turning the meat occasionally, for $2^1/_2$ to 3 hours, or until the meat is tender when pierced with a knife.

5. Strain the pan juices and skim off the fat. Slice the pork and serve it with the pan juices. Serve hot.

Lamb Chops with White Wine

Braciole di Agnello al Vino Bianco

Makes 4 servings

Here is a basic way of preparing lamb chops that can be made with either tender loin or rib cuts or chewier, but much less expensive, shoulder chops. For best flavor, trim the meat of excess fat and cook the chops just until pink in the center.

2 tablespoons olive oil

8 loin or rib lamb chops, 1 inch thick, trimmed

4 garlic cloves, lightly crushed

3 or 4 (2-inch) rosemary sprigs

Salt and freshly ground black pepper

1 cup dry white wine

1. In a skillet large enough to hold the chops comfortably in a single layer, heat the oil over medium-high heat. When the oil is hot, pat the chops dry. Sprinkle the chops with salt and pepper, then place them in the pan. Cook until the chops are browned, about 4 minutes. Scatter the garlic and rosemary around the meat. Using tongs, turn the chops and brown on the other side, about 3 minutes. Transfer the chops to a plate.

2. Add the wine to the skillet and bring to a simmer. Cook, scraping up and blending in the browned bits in the bottom of the pan, until the wine is reduced and slightly thickened, about 2 minutes.

3. Return the chops to the pan and cook them 2 minutes more, turning them in the sauce once or twice until rosy pink when cut near the bone. Transfer the chops to a platter, pour the pan juices over the chops, and serve immediately.

Lamb Chops with Capers, Lemon, and Sage

Braciole di Agnello con Capperi

Makes 4 servings

Vecchia Roma is one of my favorite Roman restaurants. On the fringe of the old ghetto, it has a beautiful outdoor garden for eating when the weather is warm and sunny, but I also enjoy the cozy inside dining rooms when it is cold or rainy. This lamb is inspired by a dish I tasted there made with tiny nuggets of baby lamb. I have adapted it to tender chops instead, because they are widely available here.

1 tablespoon olive oil

8 loin or rib lamb chops, 1 inch thick, trimmed

Salt and freshly ground black pepper

$\frac{1}{2}$ cup dry white wine

3 tablespoons fresh lemon juice

3 tablespoons capers, rinsed and chopped

6 fresh sage leaves

1. In a large skillet, heat the oil over medium-high heat. Pat the chops dry. When the oil is hot, sprinkle them with salt and pepper, then place chops in the pan. Cook until the chops are browned, about 4 minutes. Using tongs, turn the chops and brown on the other side, about 3 minutes. Transfer the chops to a plate.

2. Pour the fat out of the pan. Reduce the heat to low. Stir the wine, the lemon juice, capers, and sage into the pan. Bring to a simmer and cook 2 minutes or until slightly syrupy.

3. Return the chops to the pan and turn them once or twice until heated through and just pink when cut near the bone. Serve immediately.

Lamb Chops in Crispy Coating

Braciolette Croccante

Makes 4 servings

In Milan, I ate goat meat chops prepared this way, accompanied by artichoke hearts fried in the same crispy coating. Romans use tiny lamb chops instead of goat and leave out the cheese. Either way, a crisp mixed salad is the perfect accompaniment.

8 to 12 rib lamb chops, about ¾ inch thick, well trimmed

2 large eggs

Salt and freshly ground black pepper

1¼ cups plain dry bread crumbs

½ cup freshly grated Parmigiano-Reggiano

Olive oil for frying

1. Place the chops on a cutting board and gently pound the meat to about a ½-inch thickness.

2. In a shallow plate, beat the eggs with salt and pepper to taste. Toss the bread crumbs with the cheese on a sheet of wax paper.

3. Dip the chops one at a time in the eggs, then roll them in the bread crumbs, patting the crumbs in well.

4. Turn the oven on to the lowest setting. Pour about $^1/_2$ inch of the oil into a deep skillet. Heat the oil over medium-high heat until a little of the egg mixture cooks quickly when dropped in the oil. With tongs, carefully place a few of the chops in the oil without crowding the pan. Cook until browned and crisp, 3 to 4 minutes. Turn the chops with tongs and brown, 3 minutes. Drain the chops on paper towels. Keep the fried chops warm in the oven while frying the remainder. Serve hot.

Lamb Chops with Artichokes and Olives

Costolette di Agnello ai Carciofi e Olive

Makes 4 servings

All of the ingredients of this dish cook in the same skillet so that the complementary flavors of the lamb, artichokes, and olives blend smoothly. A bright vegetable like carrots or baked tomatoes would be a good accompaniment.

2 tablespoons olive oil

8 rib or loin lamb chops, about 1 inch thick, trimmed

Salt and freshly ground black pepper to taste

2 tablespoons olive oil

¾ cup dry white wine

8 small or 4 medium artichokes, trimmed and cut into eighths

1 garlic clove, finely chopped

½ cup small mild black olives, such as Gaeta

1 tablespoon chopped fresh flat-leaf parsley

1. In a skillet large enough to hold the chops in a single layer, heat the oil over medium heat. Pat the lamb dry. When the oil is hot, sprinkle the chops with salt and pepper, then place them in the pan. Cook until the chops are browned, 3 to 4 minutes. Using tongs, turn the chops to brown on the other side, about 3 minutes. Transfer the chops to a plate.

2. Turn the heat to medium-low. Add the wine and bring to a simmer. Cook 1 minute. Add the artichokes, garlic, and salt and pepper to taste. Cover the pan and cook 20 minutes or until the artichokes are tender.

3. Stir in the olives and parsley and cook 1 minute more. Return the chops to the pan and cook, turning the lamb once or twice until heated through. Serve immediately.

Lamb Chops with Tomato, Caper, and Anchovy Sauce

Costelette d'Agnello in Salsa

Makes 4 servings

A spicy tomato sauce flavors these Calabrese-style chops. Pork chops can also be cooked this way.

2 tablespoons olive oil

8 rib or loin lamb chops, about ¾ inch thick, trimmed

6 to 8 plum tomatoes, peeled, seeded, and chopped

4 anchovy fillets, chopped

1 tablespoon capers, rinsed and chopped

2 tablespoons chopped fresh flat-leaf parsley

1. In a skillet large enough to hold the chops comfortably in a single layer, heat the oil over medium heat. When the oil is hot, pat the chops dry. Sprinkle the chops with salt and pepper, then add the chops to the pan. Cook until the chops are browned, about 4 minutes. Using tongs, turn the chops and brown on the other side, about 3 minutes. Transfer the chops to a plate.

2. Add the tomatoes, anchovies, and capers to the pan. Add a pinch of salt and pepper to taste. Cook 5 minutes or until slightly thickened.

3. Return the chops to the pan and cook, turning them once or twice in the sauce until heated through and pink when cut near the bone. Sprinkle with parsley and serve immediately.

"Burn-the-Fingers" Lamb Chops

Agnello a Scottadito

Makes 4 servings

In the recipe that inspired this dish, from an old cookbook on Umbrian cuisine, finely chopped prosciutto fat flavors the lamb. Most cooks today substitute olive oil. Lamb riblets are also good this way.

Presumably the name comes from the idea that the chops are so delicious you can't help but eat them right away—hot, right off the grill or out of the pan.

¼ cup olive oil

2 garlic cloves, finely chopped

1 tablespoon chopped fresh rosemary

1 teaspoon chopped fresh thyme

8 rib lamb chops, about 1 inch thick, trimmed

Salt and freshly ground black pepper

1. In a small bowl, stir together the oil, garlic, herbs, and salt and pepper to taste. Brush the mixture over the lamb. Cover and refrigerate 1 hour.

2. Place a grill or broiler rack about 5 inches away from the heat source. Preheat the grill or broiler.

3. Scrape off some of the marinade. Grill or broil the chops until browned and crisp, about 5 minutes. With tongs, turn the chops over and cook until browned and just pink in the center, about 5 minutes more. Serve hot.

Grilled Lamb, Basilicata Style

Agnello allo Spiedo

Makes 4 servings

Basilicata may be best known by its portrayal in Carlo Levi's Christ Stopped at Eboli. The author painted a bleak portrait of the region before World War II, when many political prisoners were sent there in exile. Today Basilicata, though still sparsely populated, is thriving, with many tourists venturing there for the beautiful beaches near Maratea.

Pork and lamb are typical meats in this region, and the two are combined in this recipe. The pancetta wrapping around the lamb cubes gets crisp and tasty. It keeps the lamb moist and adds flavor as it grills.

$1\frac{1}{2}$ pounds boneless leg of lamb, cut into 2-inch chunks

2 garlic cloves, finely chopped

1 tablespoon chopped fresh rosemary

Salt and freshly ground black pepper

4 ounces thinly sliced pancetta

¼ cup olive oil

2 tablespoons red wine vinegar

1. Place a barbecue grill or broiler rack about 5 inches away from the heat source. Preheat the grill or broiler.

2. In a large bowl, toss the lamb with the garlic, rosemary, and salt and pepper to taste.

3. Unroll the pancetta slices. Wrap a slice of pancetta around each chunk of lamb.

4. Thread the lamb on wooden skewers, securing the pancetta in place with the skewer. Place the pieces close together without crowding. In a small bowl, whisk together the oil and vinegar. Brush the mixture over the lamb.

5. Grill or broil the skewers, turning them occasionally, until done to taste—5 to 6 minutes for medium-rare. Serve hot.

Grilled Lamb Skewers

Arrosticini

Makes 4 servings

In Abruzzo, small bites of lamb are marinated, threaded on wooden skewers, and grilled over a hot fire. The cooked skewers are served standing in a tall cup or jug, and everyone helps themselves, eating the lamb right off the sticks. They are great for a buffet, served with roasted or sautéed peppers.

2 garlic cloves

Salt

1 pound lamb from the leg, trimmed and cut into ¾-inch chunks

3 tablesoons extra-virgin olive oil

2 tablespoons chopped fresh mint

1 teaspoon chopped fresh thyme

Freshly ground black pepper

1. Chop the garlic very fine. Sprinkle the garlic with a pinch of salt and mash it with the side of a large heavy chef's knife into a fine paste.

2. In a large bowl, toss the lamb with the garlic paste, oil, herbs, and salt and pepper to taste. Cover and marinate at room temperature for 1 hour or in the refrigerator for several hours or overnight.

3. Place a barbecue grill or broiler rack about 5 inches from the heat source. Preheat the grill or broiler.

4. Thread the meat on the skewers. Place the pieces close together without crowding. Grill or broil the lamb 3 minutes or until browned. Turn the meat over with tongs and cook 2 to 3 minutes more or until browned on the outside but still pink in the center. Serve hot.

Lamb Stew with Rosemary, Mint, and White Wine

Agnello in Umido

Makes 4 servings

Lamb shoulder is ideal for stewing. The meat has enough moisture to stand up to long, slow cooking, and though tough if cooked rare, it turns out fork-tender in a stew. If only bone-in lamb shoulder is available, it can be adapted to stewing recipes. Figure on an extra pound or two of bone-in meat, depending on just how bony it is. Cook bone-in lamb about 30 minutes longer than boneless, or until the meat is coming away from the bones.

2½ pounds boneless lamb shoulder, cut into 2-inch chunks

¼ cup olive oil

Salt and freshly ground black pepper to taste

1 large onion, chopped

4 garlic cloves, chopped

2 tablespoons chopped fresh rosemary

2 tablespoons chopped fresh flat-leaf parsley

1 tablespoon chopped fresh mint

½ cup dry white wine

About ½ cup beef broth (Meat Broth) or water

2 tablespoons tomato paste

1. In a large Dutch oven or other deep, heavy pot with a tight-fitting lid, heat the oil over medium heat. Dry the lamb with paper towels. Put just as many lamb pieces as will fit comfortably in a single layer into the pot. Cook, stirring frequently, until browned on all sides, about 20 minutes. Transfer the browned lamb to a plate. Sprinkle with salt and pepper. Cook the remaining lamb in the same way.

2. When all the meat is browned, spoon off the excess fat. Add the onion, garlic, and herbs and stir well. Cook until the onion has wilted, about 5 minutes.

3. Add the wine and bring to a simmer, scraping up and blending in the browned bits on the bottom of the pot. Cook 1 minute.

4. Add the broth and tomato paste. Reduce heat to low. Cover and cook 1 hour, stirring occasionally, or until the lamb is tender. Add a little water if the sauce becomes too dry. Serve hot.

Umbrian Lamb Stew with Chickpea Puree

Agnello del Colle

Makes 6 servings

Polenta and mashed potatoes are frequent accompaniments to stews in Italy, so I was surprised when this stew was served with mashed chickpeas in Umbria. Canned chickpeas work just fine, or you can cook dried chickpeas in advance.

2 tablespoons olive oil

3 pounds boneless lamb shoulder, cut into 2-inch chunks

Salt and freshly ground black pepper

2 garlic cloves, finely chopped

1 cup dry white wine

1½ cups chopped fresh or canned tomatoes

1 (10-ounce) package white mushrooms, sliced

2 (16-ounce) cans chickpeas or 5 cups cooked chickpeas

Extra-virgin olive oil

1. In a large Dutch oven or other deep, heavy pot with a tight-fitting lid, heat the oil over medium heat. Put just enough lamb pieces in the pot as will fit comfortably in a single layer. Cook, stirring occasionally, until browned on all sides, about 20 minutes. Transfer the browned lamb to a plate. Sprinkle with salt and pepper. Cook the remaining lamb in the same way.

2. When all of the meat is browned, spoon the excess fat from the pan. Scatter the garlic in the pan and cook 1 minute. Add the wine. With a wooden spoon, scrape up and blend in to the browned bits in the bottom of the pan. Bring to a simmer and cook 1 minute.

3. Return the lamb to the pot. Add the tomatoes and mushrooms and bring to a simmer. Reduce heat to low. Cover and cook, stirring occasionally, $1^1/_2$ hours or until the lamb is tender and the sauce is reduced. If there is too much liquid, remove the cover for the last 15 minutes.

4. Just before serving, heat the chickpeas and their liquid in a medium saucepan. Then transfer them to a food processor to puree or mash them with a potato masher. Stir in a little extra-virgin olive oil and black pepper to taste. Reheat if necessary.

5. To serve, scoop some of the chickpeas onto each plate. Surround the puree with the lamb stew. Serve hot.

Hunter's-Style Lamb

Agnello alla Cacciatora

Makes 6 to 8 servings

Romans make this lamb stew with abbacchio, lamb so young that it has never eaten grass. I think the flavor of mature lamb is a better match for the zesty chopped rosemary, vinegar, garlic, and anchovy that finish the sauce.

4 pounds bone-in lamb shoulder, cut into 2-inch chunks

Salt and freshly ground black pepper

2 tablespoons olive oil

4 garlic cloves, chopped

4 fresh sage leaves

2 (2-inch) sprigs fresh rosemary

1 cup dry white wine

6 anchovy fillets

1 teaspoon finely chopped fresh rosemary leaves

2 to 3 tablespoons wine vinegar

1. Pat the pieces dry with paper towels. Sprinkle them with salt and pepper.

2. In a large Dutch oven or other deep, heavy pot with a tight-fitting lid, heat the oil over medium heat. Add just enough lamb as will fit comfortably in one layer. Cook, stirring, to brown well on all sides. Transfer the browned meat to a plate. Continue with the remaining lamb.

3. When all the lamb has been browned, spoon off most of the fat from the pan. Add half the garlic, the sage, and the rosemary, and stir. Add the wine and cook 1 minute, scraping up and blending in the browned bits on the bottom of the pan with a wooden spoon.

4. Return the lamb pieces to the pan. Reduce the heat to low. Cover and cook, stirring occasionally, for 2 hours or until the lamb is tender and coming away from the bones. Add a little water if the liquid evaporates too rapidly.

5. To make the pesto: Chop the anchovies, rosemary, and remaining garlic together. Place them in a small bowl. Stir in just enough of the vinegar to form a paste.

6. Stir the pesto into the stew and simmer 5 minutes. Serve hot.

Lamb, Potato, and Tomato Stew

Stufato di Agnello e Verdure

Makes 4 to 6 servings

Though I usually use lamb shoulder for stew, I sometimes use trimmings left over from the leg or shank. The texture of these cuts is slightly chewier, but they require less cooking and still make a good stew. Notice that in this recipe from southern Italy, the meat is put into the pot all at once, so it is only lightly browned before the other ingredients are added.

1 large onion, chopped

2 tablespoons olive oil

2 pounds boneless leg or shank of lamb, cut into 1-inch chunks

Salt and freshly ground black pepper, to taste

$\frac{1}{2}$ cup dry white wine

3 cups drained and chopped canned tomatoes

1 tablespoon chopped fresh rosemary

1 pound waxy boiling potatoes, cut into 1-inch pieces

2 carrots, cut into $\frac{1}{2}$-inch-thick slices

1 cup fresh peas or frozen peas, partially thawed

2 tablespoons chopped fresh flat-leaf parsley

1. In a large Dutch oven or other deep, heavy pot with a tight-fitting lid, cook the onion in the olive oil over medium heat until softened, about 5 minutes. Add the lamb. Cook, stirring frequently, until the pieces are lightly browned. Sprinkle with salt and pepper. Add the wine and bring it to a simmer.

2. Stir in the tomatoes and rosemary. Reduce the heat to low. Cover and cook 30 minutes.

3. Add the potatoes, carrots, and salt and pepper to taste. Simmer 30 minutes more, stirring occasionally, until the lamb and potatoes are tender. Add the peas and cook 10 minutes more. Sprinkle with parsley and serve immediately.

Lamb and Pepper Stew

Spezzato d'Agnello con Peperone

Makes 4 servings

The piquancy and sweetness of peppers and the richness of lamb make them two foods perfectly suited for each other. In this recipe, once the meat is browned, there is little to do except stir it occasionally.

$\frac{1}{4}$ cup olive oil

2 pounds boneless lamb shoulder, cut into $1\frac{1}{2}$-inch pieces

Salt and freshly ground black pepper, to taste

$\frac{1}{2}$ cup dry white wine

2 medium onions, sliced

1 large red bell pepper

1 large green bell pepper

6 plum tomatoes, peeled, seeded, and chopped

1. In a large casserole dish or Dutch oven, heat the oil over medium heat. Pat the lamb dry. Add just enough lamb to the pan as will fit comfortably in a single layer. Cook, stirring, until browned on all sides, about 20 minutes. Transfer the browned lamb to a plate. Continue cooking the remaining lamb in the same way. Sprinkle the meat all over with the salt and pepper.

2. When all the meat has been browned, spoon off excess fat. Add the wine to the pot and stir well, scraping up the browned bits. Bring to a simmer.

3. Return the lamb to the pot. Stir in the onions, peppers, and tomatoes. Reduce heat to low. Cover the pot and cook for $1^1/_2$ hours or until the meat is very tender. Serve hot.

Lamb Casserole with Eggs

Agnello Cacio e Uova

Makes 6 servings

Because eggs and lamb are both associated with springtime, it is only natural to pair them in recipes. In this dish, popular in one form or another throughout central and southern Italy, eggs and cheese form a light custardy topping on a lamb stew. It's a typical Easter recipe, so if you want to make it for the holiday meal, transfer the cooked stew to a pretty bake-and-serve casserole dish before adding the topping. A combination of lamb meat from the leg and shoulder makes for a more interesting texture.

2 tablespoons olive oil

2 medium onions

3 pounds boneless lamb leg and shoulder, trimmed and cut into 2-inch chunks

Salt and freshly ground black pepper to taste

1 tablespoon finely chopped rosemary

1½ cups homemade Meat Broth or Chicken Broth, or store-bought beef or chicken broth

2 cups shelled fresh peas or 1 (10-ounce) package frozen peas, partially thawed

3 large eggs

1 tablespoon chopped fresh flat-leaf parsley

½ cup freshly grated Pecorino Romano

1. Place a rack in the center of the oven. Preheat the oven to 425°F. In a Dutch oven or other deep, heavy pot with a tight-fitting lid, heat the oil over medium heat. Add the onion and lamb. Cook, stirring occasionally, until the lamb is lightly browned on all sides, about 20 minutes. Sprinkle with salt and pepper.

2. Add the rosemary and the broth. Stir well. Cover and bake, stirring occasionally, 60 minutes or until the meat is just tender. Add a little warm water if necessary to prevent the lamb from drying out. Stir in the peas and cook 5 minutes more.

3. In a medium bowl, beat the eggs, parsley, cheese, and salt and pepper to taste, until well blended. Pour the mixture evenly over the lamb.

4. Bake uncovered 5 minutes or until the eggs are just set. Serve immediately.

Lamb or Kid with Potatoes, Sicilian Style

Capretto o Agnello al Forno

Makes 4 to 6 servings

Baglio Elena, near Trapani in Sicily, is a working farm that produces olives, olive oil, and other foods. It is also an inn where visitors can stop for a meal in a charming, rustic dining room or stay for a vacation. When I visited, I was served a multicourse dinner of Sicilian specialties that included several types of olives prepared in different ways, excellent salame made on the premises, a variety of vegetables, and this simple stew. The meat and potatoes cook in no liquid other than a small amount of wine and the juices from the meat and vegetables, creating a symphony of flavors.

Kid is available in many ethnic butcher shops, including Haitian, Middle Eastern, and Italian. It is so similar to lamb that it can be hard to tell the difference.

3 pounds bone-in kid (young goat) or lamb shoulder, cut into 2-inch chunks

2 tablespoons olive oil

Salt and freshly ground black pepper

2 onions, thinly sliced

½ cup dry white wine

¼ teaspoon ground cloves

2 (2-inch) sprigs rosemary

1 bay leaf

4 medium all-purpose potatoes, cut into 1-inch pieces

2 cups cherry tomatoes, halved

2 tablespoons chopped fresh flat-leaf parsley

1. Place a rack in the center of the oven. Preheat the oven to 350°F. In a large Dutch oven or other deep, heavy pot with a tight-fitting lid, heat the oil over medium heat. Pat the lamb dry with paper towels. Add just enough meat to fit in the pot comfortably without crowding. Cook, turning the pieces with tongs until browned on all sides, about 15 minutes. Transfer the pieces to a plate. Continue cooking the remaining meat in the same way. Sprinkle with salt and pepper.

2. When all the meat has been browned, pour off most of the fat from the pan. Add the onion and cook, stirring occasionally, until the onion has wilted, about 5 minutes.

3. Return the meat to the pot. Add the wine and bring it to a simmer. Cook 1 minute, stirring with a wooden spoon. Add the cloves, rosemary, bay leaf, and salt and pepper to taste. Cover the pot and transfer it to the oven. Cook 45 minutes.

4. Stir in the potatoes and tomatoes. Cover and cook 45 minutes more or until the meat and potatoes are tender when pierced with a fork. Sprinkle with parsley and serve hot.

Apulian Lamb and Potato Casserole

Tiella di Agnello

Makes 6 servings

Layered casseroles baked in the oven are an Apulian specialty. They can be made with meat, fish, or vegetables, alternating with potatoes, rice, or bread crumbs. Tiella is a name given to both this method of cooking and the type of dish the casserole is cooked in. The classic tiella is a round deep dish made of terra cotta, though nowadays metal pans often are used.

The cooking method is most unusual. None of the ingredients is browned or precooked. Everything is simply layered and baked until tender. The meat will be well done, but still moist and delicious because the pieces are surrounded by the potatoes. The bottom layer of potatoes is meltingly soft and tender and full of the meat and tomato juices, while the top layer comes out as crisp as potato chips, though much more flavorful.

For the meat, use well-trimmed chunks of leg of lamb. I buy half of a butterflied leg of lamb at the supermarket, then I cut it at home into 2- to 3-inch chunks, trimming away the fat. It is just right for this recipe.

4 tablespoons olive oil

2 pounds baking potatoes, peeled and thinly sliced

$\frac{1}{2}$ cup plain dry bread crumbs

$\frac{1}{2}$ cup freshly grated Pecorino Romano or Parmigiano-Reggiano

1 garlic clove, finely chopped

$\frac{1}{2}$ cup chopped fresh flat-leaf parsley

1 tablespoon chopped fresh rosemary, or 1 teaspoon dried

$\frac{1}{2}$ teaspoon dried oregano

Salt and freshly ground black pepper

$2\frac{1}{2}$ pounds boneless lamb, trimmed and cut into 2- to 3-inch pieces

1 cup drained canned tomatoes, chopped

1 cup dry white wine

$\frac{1}{2}$ cup water

1. Place a rack in the center of the oven. Preheat the oven to 400°F. Spread 2 tablespoons of the oil in a 13 × 9 × 2–inch baking pan. Pat the potatoes dry and spread about half of them, overlapping slightly, on the bottom of the pan.

2. In a medium bowl, stir together the bread crumbs, cheese, garlic, herbs, and salt and pepper to taste. Scatter half of the crumb mixture over the potatoes. Arrange the meat on top of the crumbs. Season the meat with salt and pepper. Spread the tomatoes over the meat. Arrange the remaining potatoes on top. Pour in the wine and water. Scatter the remaining crumb mixture over all. Drizzle with the remaining 2 tablespoons olive oil.

3. Bake $1^1/_2$ to $1^3/_4$ hours or until the meat and potatoes are tender when pierced with a fork and everything is nicely browned. Serve hot.

Lamb Shanks with Chickpeas

Stinco di Agnello con Ceci

Makes 4 servings

Shanks need long, slow cooking, but when they are done, the meat is moist and just about melts in your mouth. If you purchase lamb shanks in the supermarket, the meat may need some extra trimming. With a small boning knife, cut away as much of the fat as possible, but leave intact the thin, pearly-looking covering on the meat known as the silver skin. It helps the meat to keep its shape as it cooks. I use shanks for a number of recipes that Italians would make with their smaller leg of lamb.

2 tablespoons olive oil

4 small lamb shanks, well trimmed

Salt and freshly ground black pepper

1 small onion, chopped

2 cups beef broth (Meat Broth)

1 cup peeled, seeded, and chopped tomatoes

½ teaspoon dried marjoram or thyme

4 carrots, peeled and cut into 1-inch pieces

2 tender celery ribs, cut into 1-inch chunks

3 cups cooked or 2 (16-ounce) cans chickpeas, drained

1. In a Dutch oven large enough to hold the shanks in a single layer, or another deep, heavy pot with a tight-fitting lid, heat the oil over medium heat. Pat the lamb shanks dry and brown them well on all sides, about 15 minutes. Tip the pan and spoon off the excess fat. Sprinkle with salt and pepper. Add the onion and cook 5 minutes more.

2. Add the broth, tomatoes, and marjoram and bring to a simmer. Reduce heat to low. Cover and cook 1 hour, turning the shanks occasionally.

3. Add the carrots, celery, and chickpeas. Cook 30 minutes more or until the meat is tender when pierced with a small knife. Serve hot.

Lamb Shanks with Peppers and Prosciutto

Brasato di Stinco di Agnello con Peperoni e Prosciutto

Makes 6 servings

In Senagalia, on the Adriatic coast in the Marches, I ate at the Osteria del Tempo Perso, in the historic center of this lovely old town. For a first course, I had cappelletti, stuffed "little hats" of fresh pasta with a sausage and vegetable sauce, followed by a lamb stew topped with bright-colored bell peppers and strips of prosciutto. I have adapted the flavors of the stew to lamb shanks in this recipe.

4 tablespoons olive oil

6 small lamb shanks, well trimmed

Salt and freshly ground black pepper

$1/2$ cup dry white wine

2-inch sprig fresh rosemary, or $1/2$ teaspoon dried

$1^1/_2$ cups Meat Broth

2 red bell peppers, cut into $1/_2$-inch strips

1 yellow bell pepper, cut into $1/_2$-inch strips

1 tablespoon unsalted butter

2 ounces sliced imported Italian prosciutto, cut into thin strips

2 tablespoons chopped fresh flat-leaf parsley

1. In a Dutch oven just large enough to hold the lamb shanks in a single layer, or another deep, heavy pot with a tight-fitting lid, heat the oil over medium heat. Pat the lamb shanks dry. Brown them well on all sides, turning the pieces with tongs, about 15 minutes. Tip the pan and spoon off the excess fat. Sprinkle with salt and pepper.

2. Add the wine and cook, scraping up and blending in the browned bits at the bottom of the pan with a wooden spoon. Bring to a simmer and cook 1 minute.

3. Add the rosemary and broth and bring the liquid to a simmer.

4. Partially cover the pan. Reduce heat to low. Cook, turning the meat occasionally, until the lamb is very tender when pierced with a fork, about $1^1/_4$ to $1^1/_2$ hours.

5. While the lamb is cooking, in a medium saucepan, combine the peppers, butter, and 2 tablespoons of water over medium heat. Cover and cook 10 minutes, or until the vegetables are almost tender.

6. Add the softened peppers and the prosciutto to the lamb along with the parsley. Cook uncovered over medium heat until the peppers are tender, about 5 minutes.

7. With a slotted spoon, transfer the shanks and peppers to the warmed platter. Cover and keep warm. If the liquid left in the pan is too thin, raise the heat to high and boil until reduced and slightly thickened. Taste and adjust the seasoning. Pour the sauce over the lamb and serve immediately.

Lamb Shanks with Capers and Olives

Stinchi di Agnello con Capperi e Olive

Makes 4 servings

In Sardinia, goat meat is typically used for this dish. The flavors of lamb and goat are very similar, so lamb shanks are a good substitute and are a lot easier to find.

2 tablespoons olive oil

4 small lamb shanks, well trimmed

Salt and freshly ground black pepper

1 medium onion, chopped

¾ cup dry white wine

1 cup peeled, seeded, and chopped fresh or canned tomatoes

½ cup chopped pitted black olives, such as Gaeta

2 garlic cloves, finely chopped

2 tablespoons capers, rinsed and chopped

2 tablespoons chopped fresh flat-leaf parsley

1. In a Dutch oven large enough to hold the shanks in a single layer, or another deep, heavy pot with a tight-fitting lid, heat the oil over medium heat. Pat the lamb dry and brown it well on all sides. Spoon off the excess fat. Sprinkle with salt and pepper.

2. Scatter the onion around the lamb and cook until the onion is wilted, about 5 minutes. Add the wine and cook 1 minute. Stir in the tomatoes and bring to a simmer. Reduce the heat to low and cover the pan. Cook 1 to $1^1/_2$ hours, turning the shanks occasionally, until the meat is very tender when pierced with a knife.

3. Add the olives, garlic, capers, and parsley and cook 5 minutes more, turning the meat to coat with the sauce. Serve hot.

Lamb Shanks in Tomato Sauce

Stinco di Agnello al Pomodoro

Makes 6 servings

If the only lamb shanks you can find are on the large side, you can either have the butcher split them for you, or you can cook fewer shanks, leaving them whole, then carve the meat off the bone at serving time.

6 small lamb shanks, well trimmed

2 tablespoons olive oil

2 garlic cloves, thinly sliced

1 tablespoon chopped fresh rosemary

$\frac{1}{2}$ cup dry white wine

1 cup chopped peeled tomatoes

1$\frac{1}{2}$ cups beef broth (Meat Broth)

2 tablespoons chopped fresh flat-leaf parsley

1. In a Dutch oven large enough to hold the shanks in a single layer, or another deep, heavy pot with a tight-fitting lid, heat the oil. Brown the meat on all sides, about 15 minutes. Spoon off the excess fat. Sprinkle the shanks with salt and pepper.

2. Add the garlic and rosemary to the pan and cook 1 minute. Add the wine and bring to a simmer. Add the tomatoes and broth. Reduce the heat to low, cover the pan, and cook the shanks, turning them occasionally, about $1^1/_2$ hours or until the meat is fork tender and comes away easily from the bone.

3. Sprinkle with parsley and serve hot.

Lamb Pot Roast with Cloves, Roman Style

Garofolato di Agnello

Makes 6 servings

Cloves, called chiodi di garofalo in Italian, add a distinctive flavor to this lamb pot roast from the Roman countryside. The Romans use boned and rolled lamb shoulder, but if you can't find that cut, you can substitute leg of lamb with good results.

5 whole cloves

3½ pounds boneless lamb shoulder roast, rolled and tied

Salt and freshly ground black pepper

2 tablespoons olive oil

1 medium onion, finely chopped

1 tender celery rib, finely chopped

1 carrot, chopped

¼ cup chopped fresh flat-leaf parsley

A pinch of crushed red pepper

1 cup dry white wine

2 cups tomato puree

1 cup homemade Meat Broth or canned beef broth

1. Stick the cloves into the lamb. Sprinkle the meat all over with salt and pepper.

2. In a large casserole dish or Dutch oven, heat the oil over medium heat. Add the lamb and cook, turning it with tongs, until browned on all sides, about 20 minutes.

3. Scatter the onion, celery, carrot, parsley, and red pepper around the meat. Add the wine and cook until it evaporates, about 2 minutes. Add the tomato puree and broth. Reduce the heat to low.

4. Cover and cook, turning the meat occasionally, for $2^1/_2$ to 3 hours or until tender when pierced with a fork.

5. Transfer the meat to a cutting board. Cover and keep it warm. Skim the fat from the pan juices. Pour the vegetables and pan juices into a food processor or blender and puree until smooth. Taste and adjust seasoning. Pour the sauce into a medium saucepan and reheat it over low heat. If it is too thin, simmer it until reduced. Slice the lamb and serve hot with the sauce.

Butter Rings

Bussolai

Makes 36

These Venetian cookies are simple to make and a pleasure to have around the house for a midday snack or whenever guests stop in.

1 cup sugar

$\frac{1}{2}$ cup (1 stick) unsalted butter, at room temperature

3 large egg yolks

1 teaspoon grated lemon zest

1 teaspoon grated orange zest

1 teaspoon pure vanilla extract

2 cups all-purpose flour

$\frac{1}{2}$ teaspoon salt

1 egg white, beaten until foamy

1. Set aside $\frac{1}{3}$ cup of the sugar.

2. In the large bowl of an electric mixer, beat the butter with the remaining ²/₃ cup of sugar at medium speed until light and fluffy, about 2 minutes. Beat in the egg yolks one at a time. Add the lemon and orange zests and vanilla extract and beat, scraping the sides of the bowl, until smooth, about 2 minutes more.

3. Stir in the flour and salt until well blended. Shape the dough into a ball. Wrap in plastic wrap and refrigerate 1 hour up to overnight.

4. Preheat the oven to 325°F. Grease 2 large baking sheets. Cut the dough into 6 pieces. Divide each piece again into 6 pieces. Roll each piece into a 4-inch rope, shape into a ring, and pinch the ends together to seal. Place the rings 1 inch apart on the prepared baking sheets. Brush lightly with the egg white and sprinkle with the reserved ¹/₃ cup of sugar.

5. Bake 15 minutes or until lightly browned. Have ready 2 wire cooling racks.

6. Transfer the baking sheets to the racks. Let the cookies cool 5 minutes on the baking sheets, then transfer them to the wire racks to cool completely. Store in an airtight container up to 2 weeks.

Lemon Knots

Tarralucci

Makes 40

Every Italian bakery in Brooklyn, New York, made these refreshing Sicilian lemon cookies when I was growing up. I like to serve them with iced tea.

If the weather is hot and humid, the icing may refuse to firm up at room temperature. In that case, store the cookies in the refrigerator.

4 cups all-purpose flour

4 teaspoons baking powder

1 cup sugar

½ cup solid vegetable shortening

3 large eggs

½ cup milk

2 tablespoons lemon juice

2 teaspoons grated lemon zest

Icing

1½ cups confectioner's sugar

1 tablespoon freshly squeezed lemon juice

2 teaspoons grated lemon zest

Milk

1. Sift together the flour and baking powder onto a piece of wax paper.

2. In a large bowl, with an electric mixer at medium speed, beat the sugar and shortening until light and fluffy, about 2 minutes. Beat in the eggs one at a time until well blended. Stir in the milk, lemon juice, and zest. Scrape the sides of the bowl. Stir in the dry ingredients until smooth, about 2 minutes. Cover with plastic wrap and refrigerate at least 1 hour.

3. Preheat the oven to 350°F. Have ready 2 large baking sheets. Pinch off a piece of dough the size of a golf ball. Lightly roll the dough into a 6-inch rope. Tie the rope into a knot. Place the knot on an ungreased baking sheet. Continue making the knots and placing them about 1 inch apart on the sheets.

4. Bake the cookies 12 minutes or until firm when pressed on top but not browned. Have ready 2 wire cooling racks.

5. Transfer the baking sheets to the racks. Let the cookies cool 5 minutes on the baking sheets, then transfer them to the wire racks to cool completely.

6. Combine the confectioner's sugar, lemon juice, and zest in a large bowl. Add milk 1 teaspoon at a time and stir until the mixture forms a thin icing with the consistency of heavy cream.

7. Dip the tops of the cookies in the icing. Place them on a rack until the icing is hardened. Store in airtight containers up to 3 days.

Spice Cookies

Bicciolani

Makes 75

In caffès in Turin you can order barbajada, a combination of half coffee and half hot chocolate. It would be perfect with these thin, buttery spice cookies.

1 cup (2 sticks) unsalted butter, at room temperature

1 cup sugar

1 egg yolk

2 cups all-purpose flour

$\frac{1}{2}$ teaspoon salt

1 teaspoon ground cinnamon

$\frac{1}{8}$ teaspoon freshly grated nutmeg

$\frac{1}{8}$ teaspoon ground cloves

1. Preheat the oven to 350°F. Grease a 15 × 10 × 1– inch jelly roll pan.

2. In a bowl, stir together the flour, salt, and spices.

3. In a large electric mixer bowl, beat the butter, sugar, and egg yolk on medium speed until light and fluffy, about 2 minutes. Reduce the speed to low and stir in the dry ingredients until thoroughly blended, about 2 minutes more.

4. Crumble the dough into the prepared pan. With your hands, firmly press the dough out into an even layer. With the back of a fork, make shallow ridges in the top of the dough.

5. Bake 25 to 30 minutes or until lightly browned. Transfer the pan to a wire cooling rack. Cool 10 minutes. Then cut the dough into 2 × 1–inch cookies.

6. Cool completely in the pan. Store at room temperature in an airtight container up to 2 weeks.

Wafer Cookies

Pizzelle

Makes about 2 dozen

Many families in central and southern Italy are proud of their pizzelle irons, beautifully crafted forms traditionally used to make these pretty wafers. Some irons are embossed with the original owner's initials, while others have silhouettes such as a couple toasting each other with a glass of wine. They were once a typical wedding gift.

Though charming, these old fashioned irons are heavy and unwieldy on today's stoves. An electric pizzelle press, similar to a waffle iron, does an efficient and quick job of turning out these cookies.

When they are freshly made, pizzelle are pliable and can be molded into cone, tube, or cup shapes. They can be filled with whipped cream, ice cream, cannoli cream, or fruit. They cool and crisp in no time, so you must work quickly and carefully to shape them. Of course, they are good flat as well.

1¾ cups unbleached all-purpose flour

1 teaspoon baking powder

Pinch of salt

3 large eggs

⅔ cup sugar

1 tablespoon pure vanilla extract

1 stick (½ cup) unsalted butter, melted and cooled

1. Preheat the pizzelle maker according to the manufacturer's directions. In a bowl, stir together the flour, baking powder, and salt.

2. In a large bowl, beat the eggs, sugar, and vanilla with an electric mixer on medium speed until thick and light, about 4 minutes. Beat in the butter. Stir in the dry ingredients until just blended, about 1 minute.

3. Place about 1 tablespoon of the batter in the center of each pizzelle mold. (The exact amount will depend on the design of the mold.) Close the cover and bake until lightly golden. This will depend on the maker and how long the mold has been heating. Check it carefully after 30 seconds.

4. When the pizzelle are golden, slide them off the molds with a wooden or plastic spatula. Let cool flat on a wire rack. Or, to

make cookie cups, bend each pizzelle into the curve of a wide coffee or dessert cup. To make cannoli shells, shape them around cannoli tubes or a wooden dowel.

5. When the pizzelle are cool and crisp, store them in an airtight container until ready to use. These last for several weeks.

Variation: *Anise*: Substitute 1 tablespoon anise extract and 1 tablespoon anise seeds for the vanilla. *Orange or Lemon*: Add 1 tablespoon grated fresh orange or lemon zest to the egg mixture. *Rum or Almond*: Stir in 1 tablespoon rum or almond extract instead of the vanilla. *Nut*: Stir in $1/4$ cup of nuts ground to a very fine powder along with the flour.

Sweet Ravioli

Ravioli Dolci

Makes 2 dozen

Jam fills these crisp dessert ravioli. Any flavor will do, as long as it has a thick consistency so that it will stay in place and not ooze out of the dough as it bakes. This was a favorite recipe of my father, who perfected it from his memories of the cookies his mother used to make.

1¾ cup all-purpose flour

½ cup potato or corn starch

½ teaspoon salt

½ cup (1 stick) unsalted butter, at room temperature

½ cup sugar

1 large egg

2 tablespoons rum or brandy

1 teaspoon grated lemon zest

1 teaspoon pure vanilla extract

1 cup thick sour cherry, raspberry, or apricot jam

1. In a large bowl, sift together the flour, starch, and salt.

2. In a large bowl with an electric mixer, beat the butter with the sugar until light and fluffy, about 2 minutes. Beat in the egg, rum, zest, and vanilla. On low speed, stir in the dry ingredients.

3. Divide the dough in half. Shape each half into a disk. Wrap each separately in plastic and refrigerate 1 hour up to overnight.

4. Preheat the oven to 350°F. Grease 2 large baking sheets.

5. Roll out the dough to a $1/8$-inch thickness. With a fluted pastry or pasta cutter, cut the dough into 2-inch squares. Arrange the squares about 1 inch apart on the prepared baking sheets. Place $1/2$ teaspoon of the jam in the center of each square. (Do not use more jam, or the filling will leak out as it bakes.)

6. Roll out the remaining dough to a $1/8$-inch thickness. Cut the dough into 2-inch squares.

7. Cover the jam with the dough squares. Press the edges all around with a fork to seal in the filling.

8. Bake 16 to 18 minutes, or until lightly browned. Have ready 2 wire cooling racks.

9. Transfer the baking sheets to the racks. Let the cookies cool 5 minutes on the baking sheets, then transfer them to the wire racks to cool completely. Sprinkle with confectioner's sugar. Store in an airtight container up to 1 week.

"Ugly-but-Good" Cookies

Brutti ma Buoni

Makes 2 dozen

"Ugly but good" is the meaning of the name of these Piedmontese cookies. The name is only half-true: The cookies are not ugly, but they are good. The technique for making these is unusual. The cookie batter is cooked in a saucepan before it is baked.

3 large egg whites, at room temperature

Pinch of salt

1½ cups sugar

1 cup unsweetened cocoa powder

1¼ cups hazelnuts, toasted, peeled, and coarsely chopped (see How To Toast and Skin Nuts)

1. Preheat the oven to 300°F. Grease 2 large baking sheets.

2. In a large bowl, with an electric mixer at medium speed, beat the egg whites and salt until foamy. Increase the speed to high and gradually add the sugar. Beat until soft peaks form when the beaters are lifted.

3. On low speed, mix in the cocoa. Stir in the hazelnuts.

4. Scrape the mixture into a large heavy saucepan. Cook over medium heat, stirring constantly with a wooden spoon, until the mixture is shiny and smooth, about 5 minutes. Be careful that it does not scorch.

5. Immediately drop the hot batter by tablespoonfuls onto the prepared baking sheets. Bake 30 minutes or until firm and slightly cracked on the surface.

6. While the cookies are still hot, transfer them to a rack to cool, using a thin-blade metal spatula. Store in an airtight container up to 2 weeks.

Jam Spots

Biscotti di Marmellata

Makes 40

Chocolate, nuts, and jam are a winning combination in these tasty cookies. They are always a hit on Christmas cookie trays.

¾ cup (1½ sticks) unsalted butter, at room temperature

½ cup sugar

½ teaspoon salt

3 ounces bittersweet chocolate, melted and cooled

2 cups all-purpose flour

¾ cup finely chopped almonds

½ cup thick seedless raspberry jam

1. Preheat the oven to 350°F. Grease 2 large baking sheets.

2. In a large bowl, with an electric mixer on medium speed, beat the butter, sugar, and salt until light and fluffy, about 2 minutes.

Add the melted chocolate and beat until well blended, scraping the sides of the bowl. Stir in the flour until smooth.

3. Place the nuts in a shallow bowl. Shape the dough into 1-inch balls. Roll the balls in the nuts, pressing lightly so they will adhere. Place the balls about $1^1/_2$ inches apart on the prepared baking sheets.

4. With the handle end of a wooden spoon, poke a deep hole in each ball of dough, molding the dough around the handle to maintain the round shape. Place about $^1/_4$ teaspoon jam in each cookie. (Do not add more jam, as it may melt and leak out when the cookies bake.)

5. Bake the cookies 18 to 20 minutes, or until the jam is bubbling and the cookies are lightly browned. Have ready 2 wire cooling racks.

6. Transfer the baking sheets to the racks. Let the cookies cool 5 minutes on the baking sheets, then transfer them to the wire racks to cool completely. Store in an airtight container up to 2 weeks.

Double-Chocolate Nut Biscotti

Biscotti al Cioccolato

Makes 4 dozen

These rich biscotti have chocolate in the dough, both melted and in chunks. I have never seen them in Italy, but they are similar to what I have tasted in coffee bars here.

2½ cups all-purpose flour

2 teaspoons baking powder

½ teaspoon salt

3 large eggs, at room temperature

1 cup sugar

1 teaspoon pure vanilla extract

6 ounces bittersweet chocolate, melted and cooled

6 tablespoons (½ stick plus 2 tablespoons) unsalted butter, melted and cooled

1 cup walnuts, coarsely chopped

1 cup chocolate chips

1. Place a rack in the center of the oven. Preheat the oven to 300°F. Grease and flour 2 large baking sheets.

2. In a large bowl, sift together the flour, baking powder, and salt.

3. In a large bowl, with an electric mixer at medium speed, beat the eggs, sugar, and vanilla until foamy and light, about 2 minutes. Stir in the chocolate and butter until blended. Add the flour mixture and stir until smooth, about 1 minute more. Stir in the nuts and chocolate chips.

4. Divide the dough in half. With moistened hands, shape each piece into a 12 × 3–inch log on the prepared baking sheet. Bake for 35 minutes or until the logs are firm when pressed in the center. Remove the pan from the oven, but do not turn off the heat. Let cool 10 minutes.

5. Slide the logs onto a cutting board. Cut the logs into $1/2$-inch-thick slices. Lay the slices on the baking sheet. Bake for 10 minutes or until the cookies are lightly toasted.

6. Have ready 2 large cooling racks. Transfer the baking sheets to the racks. Let the cookies cool 5 minutes on the baking sheets, then transfer them to the racks to cool completely. Store in an airtight container up to 2 weeks.

Chocolate Kisses

Baci di Cioccolato

Makes 3 dozen

Chocolate and vanilla "kisses" are a favorite in Verona, home of Romeo and Juliet, where they are made in a variety of combinations.

1²/₃ cups all-purpose flour

¹/₃ cup unsweetened Dutch-process cocoa powder, sifted

¹/₄ teaspoon salt

1 cup (2 sticks) unsalted butter, at room temperature

¹/₂ cup confectioner's sugar

1 teaspoon pure vanilla extract

¹/₂ cup finely chopped toasted almonds (see How To Toast and Skin Nuts)

Filling

2 ounces semisweet or bittersweet chocolate, chopped

2 tablespoons unsalted butter

⅓ cup almonds, toasted and finely chopped

1. In a large bowl, sift together the flour, cocoa, and salt.

2. In a large bowl, with an electric mixer at medium speed, beat the butter and sugar until light and fluffy, about 2 minutes. Beat in the vanilla. Stir in the dry ingredients and the almonds until blended, about 1 minute more. Cover with plastic and chill in the refrigerator 1 hour up to overnight.

3. Preheat the oven to 350°F. Have ready 2 ungreased baking sheets. Roll teaspoonfuls of the dough into ³/₄-inch balls. Place the balls 1 inch apart on the baking sheets. With your fingers, press the balls to flatten them slightly. Bake the cookies until firm but not browned, 10 to 12 minutes. Have ready 2 large cooling racks.

4. Transfer the baking sheets to the racks. Let the cookies cool 5 minutes on the baking sheets, then transfer them to the racks to cool completely.

5. Bring about 2 inches of water to a simmer in the bottom half of a double boiler or a small saucepan. Place the chocolate and the butter in the top half of the double boiler or in a small heatproof bowl that fits comfortably over the saucepan. Place the bowl over the simmering water. Let stand uncovered until the chocolate is softened. Stir until smooth. Stir in the almonds.

6. Spread a small amount of the filling mixture on the bottom of one cookie. Place a second cookie bottom-side down on the filling and press together lightly. Place the cookies on a wire rack until the filling is set. Repeat with the remaining cookies and filling. Store in an airtight container in the refrigerator up to 1 week.

No-Bake Chocolate "Salame"

Salame del Cioccolato

Makes 32 cookies

Crunchy chocolate nut slices that require no baking are a specialty of Piedmont. Other cookies can be substituted for the amaretti, if you prefer, such as vanilla or chocolate wafers, graham crackers, or shortbread. These are best made a few days ahead, to allow the flavors to blend. If you prefer not use the liqueur, substitute a spoonful of orange juice.

18 amaretti cookies

$\frac{1}{3}$ cup sugar

$\frac{1}{3}$ cup unsweetened cocoa powder

$\frac{1}{2}$ cup (1 stick) unsalted butter, softened

1 tablespoon grappa or rum

$\frac{1}{3}$ cup chopped walnuts

1. Place the cookies in a plastic bag. Crush the cookies with a rolling pin or heavy object. There should be about $\frac{3}{4}$ cup of crumbs.

2. Place the crumbs in a large bowl. With a wooden spoon, stir in the sugar and cocoa. Add the butter and grappa. Stir until the dry ingredients are moistened and blended. Stir in the walnuts.

3. Place a 14-inch sheet of plastic wrap on a flat surface. Pour the dough mixture onto the plastic wrap. Shape the dough into an 8 × 2^1/$_2$–inch log. Roll the log in the plastic wrap, folding the ends over to enclose it completely. Refrigerate the log at least 24 hours and up to 3 days.

4. Cut the log into ^{1}/$_4$-inch-thick slices. Serve chilled. Store the cookies in an airtight plastic container in the refrigerator up to 2 weeks.

Prato Biscuits

Biscotti di Prato

Makes about 4½ dozen

In the town of Prato in Tuscany, these are the classic biscotti to dip in vin santo, the great dessert wine of the region. Eaten plain, they are rather dry, so do provide a beverage for dunking them.

2½ cups all-purpose flour

1½ teaspoons baking powder

1 teaspoon salt

4 large eggs

¾ cup sugar

1 teaspoon grated lemon zest

1 teaspoon grated orange zest

1 teaspoon pure vanilla extract

1 cup toasted almonds (see How To Toast and Skin Nuts)

1. Place a rack in the center of the oven. Preheat the oven to 325°F. Grease and flour a large baking sheet.

2. In a medium bowl, sift together the flour, baking powder, and salt.

3. In a large bowl with an electric mixer, beat the eggs and sugar on medium speed until light and foamy, about 3 minutes. Beat in the lemon and orange zests and vanilla. On low speed, stir in the dry ingredients, then stir in the almonds.

4. Lightly dampen your hands. Shape the dough into two 14 × 2–inch logs. Place the logs on the prepared baking sheet several inches apart. Bake for 30 minutes or until firm and golden.

5. Remove the baking sheet from the oven and reduce the oven heat to 300°F. Let the logs cool on the baking sheet for 20 minutes.

6. Slide the logs onto a cutting board. With a large heavy chef's knife, cut the logs on the diagonal into $1/2$-inch-thick slices. Lay the slices on the baking sheet. Bake 20 minutes or until lightly golden.

7. Transfer the cookies to wire racks to cool. Store in an airtight container.

Umbrian Fruit and Nut Biscotti

Tozzetti

Makes 80

Made without fat, these cookies keep a long time in an airtight container. The flavor actually improves, so plan to make them several days before serving them.

3 cups all-purpose flour

½ cup cornstarch

2 teaspoons baking powder

3 large eggs

3 egg yolks

2 tablespoons Marsala, vin santo, or sherry

1 cup sugar

1 cup raisins

1 cup almonds

¼ cup chopped candied orange peel

¼ cup chopped candied citron

1 teaspoon anise seeds

1. Preheat the oven to 350°F. Grease 2 large baking sheets.

2. In a medium bowl, sift together the flour, cornstarch, and baking powder.

3. In a large bowl with an electric mixer, beat together the eggs, yolks, and Marsala. Add the sugar and beat until well blended, about 3 minutes. Stir in the dry ingredients, the raisins, almonds, peel, citron and anise seeds until blended. The dough will be stiff. If necessary, turn the dough out onto a countertop and knead it until blended.

4. Divide the dough into quarters. Dampen your hands with cool water and shape each quarter into a 10-inch log. Place the logs 2 inches apart on the prepared baking sheets.

5. Bake the logs 20 minutes or until they feel firm when pressed in the center and are golden brown around the edges. Remove the logs from the oven but leave the oven on. Let the logs cool 5 minutes on the baking sheets.

6. Slide the logs onto a cutting board. With a large chef's knife, cut them into $1/2$-inch-thick slices. Place the slices on the baking sheets and bake 10 minutes or until lightly toasted.

7. Have ready 2 large cooling racks. Transfer the cookies to the racks. Let cool completely. Store in an airtight container up to 2 weeks.

Lemon Nut Biscotti

Biscotti al Limone

Makes 48

Lemon and almonds flavor these biscotti.

1½ cups all-purpose flour

1 teaspoon baking powder

¼ teaspoon salt

½ cup (1 stick) unsalted butter, at room temperature

½ cup sugar

2 large eggs, at room temperature

2 teaspoons freshly grated lemon zest

1 cup toasted almonds, coarsely chopped

1. Place a rack in the center of the oven. Preheat the oven to 350°F. Grease and flour a large baking sheet.

2. In a bowl, sift together the flour, baking powder, and salt.

3. In a large bowl with an electric mixer, beat the butter and sugar until light and fluffy, about 2 minutes. Beat in the eggs one at a time. Add the lemon zest, scraping the inside of the bowl with a rubber spatula. Gradually stir in the flour mixture and the nuts until blended.

4. Divide the dough in half. With moistened hands, shape each piece into a 12 × 2–inch log on the prepared baking sheet. Bake for 20 minutes or until the logs are lightly browned and firm when pressed in the center. Remove the pan from the oven, but do not turn off the heat. Let the logs cool 10 minutes on the baking sheet.

5. Slide the logs onto a cutting board. Cut the logs into $^1/_2$-inch-thick slices. Place the slices on the baking sheet. Bake for 10 minutes or until the cookies are lightly toasted.

6. Have ready 2 large cooling racks. Transfer the cookies to the racks. Let cool completely. Store in an airtight container up to 2 weeks.

Walnut Biscotti

Biscotti di Noce

Makes about 80

Olive oil can be used for baking in a wide range of recipes. Use a mild-flavored extra-virgin olive oil. It complements many types of nuts and citrus fruits. Here is a biscotti recipe I developed for an article in the Washington Post about baking with olive oil.

2 cups all-purpose flour

1 teaspoon baking powder

1 teaspoon salt

2 large eggs, at room temperature

⅔ cup sugar

½ cup extra-virgin olive oil

½ teaspoon grated lemon zest

2 cups toasted walnuts (see How To Toast and Skin Nuts)

1. Preheat the oven to 325°F. Grease 2 large baking sheets.

2. In a large bowl, combine the flour, baking powder, and salt.

3. In another large bowl, whisk the eggs, sugar, oil, and lemon zest until well blended. With a wooden spoon, stir in the dry ingredients just until blended. Stir in the walnuts.

4. Divide the dough into four pieces. Shape the pieces into 12 × $1^1/_2$–inch logs, placing them several inches apart on the prepared baking sheets. Bake for 20 to 25 minutes or until lightly browned. Remove from the oven, but do not turn it off. Let the cookies cool on the baking sheets 10 minutes.

5. Slide the logs onto a cutting board. With a large heavy knife, cut the logs diagonally into $^1/_2$-inch slices. Lay the slices on the baking sheets and return the sheets to the oven. Bake 10 minutes or until toasted and golden.

6. Have ready 2 large cooling racks. Transfer the cookies to the racks. Let cool completely. Store in an airtight container up to 2 weeks.

Almond Macaroons

Amaretti

Makes 3 dozen

In southern Italy, these are made by grinding up both sweet and bitter almonds. Bitter almonds, which come from a particular variety of almond tree, are not sold in the United States. They have a flavor component similar to cyanide, a lethal poison, so they are not approved for commercial use. The closest we can come to the correct flavor is commercial almond paste and a little almond extract. Do not confuse almond paste with marzipan, which is similar, but has a higher sugar content. Buy the almond paste sold in cans for best flavor. If you can't find it, ask at your local bakery to see if they will sell you some.

These cookies stick, so I bake them on nonstick baking mats known as Silpat. The mats never need greasing, are easy to clean, and reusable. You can find them at good kitchen supply stores. If you don't have the mats, the baking pans can be lined with parchment paper or aluminum foil.

1 (8-ounce) can almond paste, crumbled

1 cup sugar

2 large egg whites, at room temperature

$\frac{1}{4}$ teaspoon almond extract

36 candied cherries or whole almonds

1. Preheat the oven to 350°F. Line 2 large baking sheets with parchment paper or aluminum foil.

2. Crumble the almond paste into a large bowl. With an electric mixer on low speed, beat in the sugar until blended. Add the egg whites and almond extract. Increase the speed to medium and beat until very smooth, about 3 minutes.

3. Scoop up 1 tablespoon of the batter and lightly roll it into a ball. Dampen your fingertips with cool water if necessary to prevent sticking. Place the balls about one inch apart on the prepared baking sheet. Press a cherry or almond into the top of the dough.

4. Bake 18 to 20 minutes or until the cookies are lightly browned. Let cool briefly on the baking sheet.

5. With a thin metal spatula, transfer the cookies to wire racks to cool completely. Store the cookies in airtight containers. (If you want to keep these cookies for more than a day or two, freeze

them to maintain their soft texture. They can be eaten directly from the freezer.)

Pine Nut Macaroons

Biscotti di Pinoli

Makes 40

I have made many variations of these cookies over the years. This version is my favorite because it is made with both almond paste and ground almonds for both flavor and texture and has the added rich flavor of toasted pine nuts (pignoli).

1 (8-ounce) can almond paste

⅓ cup finely ground blanched almonds

2 large egg whites

1 cup confectioner's sugar, plus more for decorating

2 cups pine nuts or slivered almonds

1. Place a rack in the center of the oven. Preheat the oven to 350°F. Grease a large baking sheet.

2. In a large bowl, crumble the almond paste. With an electric mixer on medium speed, beat in the almonds, egg whites, and 1 cup of confectioner's sugar until smooth.

3. Scoop up a tablespoon of the batter. Roll the batter in the pine nuts, covering it completely and forming a ball. Place the ball on the prepared baking sheet. Repeat with the remaining ingredients, placing the balls about 1 inch apart.

4. Bake 18 to 20 minutes or until lightly browned. Place the baking sheet on a cooling rack. Let the cookies cool 2 minutes on the baking sheet.

5. Transfer the cookies to racks to cool completely. Dust with confectioner's sugar. Store in an airtight container in the refrigerator up to 1 week.

Hazelnut Bars

Nocciolate

Makes 6 dozen

These tender, crumbly bars are packed with nuts. They barely hold together and melt in the mouth. Serve them with chocolate ice cream.

2 ⅓ cups all-purpose flour

1½ cups peeled, toasted hazelnuts, finely chopped (see How To Toast and Skin Nuts)

1½ cups sugar

½ teaspoon salt

1 cup (2 sticks) unsalted butter, melted and cooled

1 large egg plus 1 egg yolk, beaten

1. Place a rack in the center of the oven. Preheat the oven to 350°F. Grease a 15 × 10 × 1–inch jelly roll pan.

2. In a large bowl with a wooden spoon, stir together the flour, nuts, sugar, and salt. Add the butter and stir until evenly moistened. Add the eggs. Stir until well blended and the mixture holds together.

3. Pour the mixture into the prepared pan. Firmly pat it out into an even layer.

4. Bake 30 minutes or until golden brown. While still hot, cut into 2 × 1–inch rectangles.

5. Let cool 10 minutes in the pan. Transfer the cookies to large racks to cool completely.

Walnut Butter Cookies

Biscotti di Noce

Makes 5 dozen

Nutty and buttery, these crescent-shaped cookies from Piedmont are perfect for Christmas. Though they are often made with hazelnuts, I like to use walnuts. Almonds can also be substituted.

These cookies can be made entirely in the food processor. If you don't have one, grind the nuts and sugar in a blender or nut grinder, then stir in the remaining ingredients by hand.

1 cup walnut pieces

⅓ cup sugar plus 1 cup more for rolling the cookies

2 cups all-purpose flour

1 cup (2 sticks) unsalted butter, at room temperature

1. Preheat oven to 350°F. Grease and flour 2 large baking sheets.

2. In a food processor, combine the walnuts and sugar. Process until the nuts are finely chopped. Add the flour and process until blended.

3. Add the butter a little at a time and pulse to blend. Remove the dough from the container and squeeze it together with your hands.

4. Pour the remaining 1 cup of sugar into a shallow bowl. Pinch off a piece of dough the size of a walnut and form it into a ball. Shape the ball into a crescent, tapering the ends. Gently roll the crescent in sugar. Place the crescent on a prepared baking sheet. Repeat with the remaining dough and sugar, placing each cookie about 1 inch apart.

5. Bake 15 minutes or until lightly browned. Place the baking sheets on wire racks to cool 5 minutes.

6. Transfer the cookies to the racks to cool completely. Store in an airtight container up to 2 weeks.

Rainbow Cookies

Biscotti Tricolori

Makes about 4 dozen

Though I have never seen them in Italy, these "rainbow," or tricolored, cookies with a chocolate glaze are a favorite at Italian and other bakeries in the United States. Unfortunately, they are often colored garishly and can be dry and tasteless.

Try this recipe and you will see how good these cookies can be. They are a bit fussy to make, but the results are very pretty and delicious. If you prefer not to use food coloring, the cookies will still be attractive. For convenience, it is best to have three identical baking pans. But you can still make the cookies with only one pan if you bake one batch of dough at a time. The finished cookies keep well in the refrigerator.

8 ounces almond paste

1½ cups (3 sticks) unsalted butter

1 cup sugar

4 large eggs, separated

¼ teaspoon salt

2 cups unbleached all-purpose flour

10 drops red food coloring, or to taste (optional)

10 drops green food coloring, or to taste (optional)

½ cup apricot preserves

½ cup seedless raspberry jam

1 (6-ounce) package semisweet chocolate chips

1. Preheat the oven to 350°F. Grease three 13 × 9 × 2– inch identical baking pans. Line the pans with wax paper and grease the paper.

2. Crumble the almond paste into a large mixer bowl. Add the butter, $1/2$ cup of the sugar, the egg yolks, and salt. Beat until light and fluffy. Stir in the flour just until blended.

3. In another large bowl, with clean beaters, beat the egg whites on medium speed until foamy. Gradually beat in the remaining sugar. Increase the speed to high. Continue beating until the egg whites form soft peaks when the beaters are lifted.

4. With a rubber spatula, fold $^1/_3$ of the whites into the yolk mixture to lighten it. Gradually fold in the remaining whites.

5. Scoop $^1/_3$ of the batter into one bowl, and another $^1/_3$ into another bowl. If using the food coloring, fold the red into one bowl and the green into the other.

6. Spread each bowl of batter into a separate prepared pan, smoothing it out evenly with a spatula. Bake the layers 10 to 12 minutes, until the cake is just set and very lightly colored around the edges. Let cool in the pan for 5 minutes, then lift the layers onto cooling racks, leaving the wax paper attached. Let cool completely.

7. Using the paper to lift one layer, invert the cake and place it paper-side up on a large tray. Carefully peel off the paper. Spread with a thin layer of the raspberry jam.

8. Set a second layer paper-side up on top of the first. Remove the paper and spread the cake with the apricot jam.

9. Place the remaining layer paper-side up on top. Peel off the paper. With a large heavy knife and a ruler as a guide, trim the edges of the cake to make the layers straight and even all around.

10. Bring about 2 inches of water to a simmer in the bottom half of a double boiler or a small saucepan. Place the chocolate chips in the top half of the double boiler or in a small heatproof bowl that fits comfortably over the saucepan. Place the bowl over the simmering water. Let stand uncovered until the chocolate is softened. Stir until smooth. Pour the melted chocolate on top of the cake layers and spread it smooth with a spatula. Refrigerate until the chocolate is just beginning to set, about 30 minutes. (Don't let it get too hard, or it will crack when you cut it.)

11. Remove the cake from the refrigerator. Using a ruler or other straight edge as a guide, cut the cake lengthwise into 6 strips by first cutting it into thirds, then cutting each third in half. Cut crosswise into 5 strips. Chill the cut cake in the pan in the refrigerator until the chocolate is firm. Serve or transfer the cookies to an airtight container and store in the refrigerator. These keep well for several weeks.

Christmas Fig Cookies

Cuccidati

Makes 18 large cookies

I can't imagine Christmas without these cookies. For many Sicilians, making them is a family project. The women mix and roll the dough, while the men chop and grind the filling ingredients. The children decorate the filled cookies. They are traditionally cut into many fanciful shapes resembling birds, leaves, or flowers. Some families make dozens of them to give away to friends and neighbors.

Dough

2½ cups all-purpose flour

⅓ cup sugar

2 teaspoons baking powder

½ teaspoon salt

6 tablespoons unsalted butter

2 large eggs, at room temperature

1 teaspoon pure vanilla extract

Filling

2 cups moist dried figs, stems removed

½ cup raisins

1 cup walnuts, toasted and chopped

½ cup chopped semisweet chocolate (about 2 ounces)

⅓ cup honey

¼ cup orange juice

1 teaspoon orange zest

1 teaspoon ground cinnamon

⅛ teaspoon ground cloves

Assembly

1 egg yolk beaten with 1 teaspoon water

Colored candy sprinkles

1. Prepare the dough: In a large bowl, combine the flour, sugar, baking powder, and salt. Cut in the butter, using an electric mixer or pastry blender, until the mixture resembles coarse crumbs.

2. In a bowl, whisk the eggs and vanilla. Add the eggs to the dry ingredients, stirring with a wooden spoon until the dough is evenly moistened. If the dough is too dry, blend in a little cold water a few drops at a time.

3. Gather the dough into a ball and place it on a sheet of plastic wrap. Flatten it into a disk and wrap well. Refrigerate at least 1 hour or overnight.

4. Prepare the filling: In a food processor or meat grinder, grind the figs, raisins, and nuts until coarsely chopped. Stir in the remaining ingredients. Cover and refrigerate if not using within the hour.

5. To assemble the pastries, preheat the oven to 375°F. Grease two large baking sheets.

6. Cut the dough into 6 pieces. On a lightly floured surface, roll each piece into a log about 4 inches long.

7. With a floured rolling pin, roll one log into a 9 × 5-inch rectangle. Trim the edges.

8. Spoon a $3/4$-inch strip of the filling lengthwise slightly to one side of the center of the rolled out dough. Fold one long side of the dough over to the other and press the edges together to seal. Cut the filled dough crosswise into 3 even pieces.

9. With a sharp knife, cut slits $3/4$-inch long at $1/2$-inch intervals through the filling and dough. Curving them slightly to open the slits and reveal the fig filling, place the pastries one inch apart on the baking sheets.

10. Brush the pastry with the egg wash. Drizzle with candy sprinkles if desired. Repeat with the remaining ingredients.

11. Bake the cookies 20 to 25 minutes or until golden brown.

12. Cool the cookies on wire racks. Store in an airtight container in the refrigerator up to 1 month.

Almond Brittle

Croccante or Torrone

Makes 10 to 12 servings

Sicilians make these sweets with pine nuts, pistachios, or sesame seeds in place of the almonds. A lemon is perfect to smooth out the hot syrup.

Vegetable oil

2 cups sugar

¼ cup honey

2 cups almonds (10 ounces)

1 whole lemon, washed and dried

1. Brush a marble surface or a metal baking sheet with neutral-flavored vegetable oil.

2. In a medium saucepan, combine the sugar and honey. Cook over medium-low heat, stirring occasionally, until the sugar begins to melt, about 20 minutes. Bring to a simmer and cook without stirring 5 minutes more or until the syrup is clear.

3. Add the nuts and cook until the syrup is amber-colored, about 3 minutes. Carefully pour the hot syrup onto the prepared surface, using the lemon to smooth the nuts to a single layer. Let cool completely. When the brittle is cool and hard, after about 30 minutes, slide a thin metal spatula underneath it. Lift the brittle and break it into $1^1/_2$-inch pieces. Store in airtight containers at room temperature.

Sicilian Nut Rolls

Mostaccioli

Makes 64 cookies

At one time these cookies were made with mosto cotto, concentrated wine grape juice. Today's cooks use honey.

Dough

3 cups all-purpose flour

$\frac{1}{2}$ cup sugar

1 teaspoon salt

$\frac{1}{2}$ cup shortening

4 tablespoons ($\frac{1}{2}$ stick) unsalted butter, at room temperature

2 large eggs

2 to 3 tablespoons cold milk

Filling

1 cup toasted almonds

1 cup toasted walnuts

½ cup toasted and skinned hazelnuts

¼ cup sugar

¼ cup honey

2 teaspoons orange zest

¼ teaspoon ground cinnamon

Confectioner's sugar

1. In a large bowl, combine the flour, sugar, and salt. Cut in the shortening and butter until the mixture resembles coarse crumbs.

2. In a small bowl, whisk the eggs with two tablespoons of the milk. Add the mixture to the dry ingredients, stirring until the dough is evenly moistened. If needed, blend in a little more milk.

3. Gather the dough into a ball and place it on a sheet of plastic wrap. Flatten it into a disk and wrap well. Refrigerate 1 hour up to overnight.

4. Process the nuts and sugar in a food processor. Process until fine. Add the honey, zest, and cinnamon, and process until

blended. Preheat the oven to 350°F. Grease 2 large baking sheets.

5. Divide the dough into 4 pieces. Roll out one piece between two sheets of plastic wrap to form a square slightly larger than 8 inches. Trim the edges and cut the dough into 2-inch squares. Place a heaping teaspoon of the filling along one side of each square. Roll up the dough to enclose the filling completely. Place seam-side down on the baking pan. Repeat with the remaining dough and filling, placing the cookies 1 inch apart.

6. Bake 18 minutes or until the cookies are lightly browned. Transfer the cookies to wire racks to cool. Store in a tightly sealed container up to 2 weeks. Sprinkle with confectioner's sugar before serving.

Sponge Cake

Pan di Spagna

Makes two 8- or 9-inch layers

This classic and versatile Italian sponge cake works well with fillings such as fruit preserves, whipped cream, pastry cream, ice cream, or ricotta cream. The cake also freezes well, so it is convenient to have on hand for quick desserts.

Butter for the pan

6 large eggs, at room temperature

$\frac{2}{3}$ cup sugar

1$\frac{1}{2}$ teaspoons pure vanilla extract

1 cup sifted all-purpose flour

1. Place the rack in the center of the oven. Preheat the oven to 375°F. Butter two 8- or 9-inch layer cake pans. Line the bottom of the pans with circles of waxed paper or parchment paper. Butter the paper. Dust the pans with flour and tap out the excess.

2. In a large bowl with an electric mixer, begin beating the eggs on low speed. Slowly add the sugar, gradually increasing the mixer speed to high. Add the vanilla. Beat the eggs until thick and pale yellow, about 7 minutes.

3. Place the flour in a fine-mesh strainer. Shake about one-third of the flour over the egg mixture. Gradually and very gently fold in the flour with a rubber spatula. Repeat, adding the flour in 2 additions and folding it in until there are no streaks.

4. Spread the batter evenly in the prepared pans. Bake 20 to 25 minutes or until the cakes spring back when pressed lightly in the center and the top is lightly browned. Have ready 2 cooling racks. Cool the cakes 10 minutes in the pans on the wire racks.

5. Invert the cakes onto the racks and remove the pans. Carefully peel off the paper. Let cool completely. Serve immediately or cover with an inverted bowl and store at room temperature up to 2 days.

Citrus Sponge Cake

Torta di Agrumi

Serves 10 to 12

Olive oil gives this cake a distinctive flavor and texture. Use a mild olive oil or the flavor could be intrusive. Because it does not contain butter, milk, or other dairy products, this cake is good for people who cannot eat those foods.

This is a big cake, though it is very light and airy. To bake it, you will need a 10-inch tube pan with a removable bottom—the kind used for angel cakes.

A little bit of cream of tartar, available in the spice section of most supermarkets, helps to stabilize the egg whites in this large cake.

2¼ cups plain cake flour (not self-rising)

1 tablespoon baking powder

1 teaspoon salt

6 large eggs, separated, at room temperature

1¼ cups sugar

1½ teaspoons orange zest

1½ teaspoons grated lemon zest

¾ cup freshly squeezed orange juice

½ cup extra-virgin olive oil

1 teaspoon pure vanilla extract

¼ teaspoon cream of tartar

1. Place the oven rack in the lower third of the oven. Preheat the oven to 325°F. In a large bowl, sift together the flour, baking powder, and salt.

2. In a large bowl with an electric mixer, beat the egg yolks, 1 cup of the sugar, the orange and lemon zests, the orange juice, oil, and vanilla extract until smooth, about 5 minutes. With a rubber spatula, fold the liquid into the dry ingredients.

3. In another large bowl with clean beaters, beat the egg whites on medium speed until foamy. Gradually add the remaining ¹/₄ cup of sugar and the cream of tartar. Increase the speed to high. Beat until soft peaks form when the beaters are lifted, about 5 minutes. Fold the whites into the batter.

4. Scrape the batter into an ungreased 10-inch tube pan with a removable bottom. Bake 55 minutes or until the cake is golden brown and a toothpick inserted in the center comes out clean.

5. Place the pan upside down on a cooling rack and let the cake cool completely. Run a thin-blade knife around the inside of the pan to loosen the cake. Lift out the cake and the bottom of the pan. Slide the knife under the cake and remove the pan bottom. Serve immediately, or cover with an overturned bowl and store at room temperature up to 2 days.

Lemon Olive-Oil Cake

Torta di Limone

Makes 8 servings

A light, lemony cake from Puglia that is always a pleasure to have on hand.

1½ cups plain cake flour (not self-rising)

1½ teaspoons baking powder

½ teaspoon salt

3 large eggs, at room temperature

1 cup sugar

⅓ cup olive oil

1 teaspoon pure vanilla extract

1 teaspoon grated lemon zest

¼ cup freshly squeezed lemon juice

1. Place the rack in the lowest third of the oven. Preheat oven to 350°F. Grease a 9-inch springform pan.

2. In a large bowl, sift together the flour, baking powder, and salt.

3. Break the eggs into a large electric mixer bowl. Beat on medium speed until thick and pale yellow, about 5 minutes. Slowly add in the sugar and beat 3 minutes more. Slowly add the oil. Beat one minute more. Add the vanilla and lemon zest.

4. With a rubber spatula, fold in the dry ingredients in three additions, alternating with the lemon juice in two additions.

5. Scrape the batter into the prepared pan. Bake 35 to 40 minutes or until the cake is golden brown and springs back when pressed in the center.

6. Turn the pan upside down on a wire rack. Let cool completely. Run a knife around the outside rim and remove it. Serve immediately, or cover with an overturned bowl and store at room temperature up to 2 days.

Marble Cake

Torta Marmorata

Makes 8 to 10 servings

Breakfast is not given a lot of attention in Italy. Eggs and cereal are rarely eaten, and most Italians get by on coffee with toast or perhaps a plain cookie or two. Hotel breakfasts often overcompensate for foreign tastes with a lavish variety of cold meats, cheeses, fruit, eggs, yogurt, bread, and pastries. At one hotel in Venice, I spotted a magnificent marble cake, one of my personal favorite cakes, proudly displayed on a cake stand. It was heavenly with a cup of cappuccino, and I would have enjoyed it equally at teatime. The waiter told me the cake was delivered fresh daily from a local bakery where it was a specialty. This is my version, inspired by the one in Venice.

1½ cups plain cake flour (not self-rising)

1½ teaspoons baking powder

½ teaspoon salt

3 large eggs, at room temperature

1 cup sugar

$\frac{1}{3}$ cup vegetable oil

1 teaspoon pure vanilla extract

$\frac{1}{4}$ teaspoon almond extract

$\frac{1}{2}$ cup milk

2 ounces bittersweet or semisweet chocolate, melted and cooled

1. Place the oven rack in the lowest third of the oven. Preheat the oven to 325°F. Grease and flour a 10-inch tube pan and tap out the excess flour.

2. In a large bowl, sift together the flour, baking powder, and salt.

3. In another large bowl, with an electric mixer, beat the eggs on medium speed until thick and pale yellow, about 5 minutes. Slowly beat in the sugar a tablespoon at a time. Continue beating 2 minutes more.

4. Gradually beat in the oil and extracts. Fold in the flour in 3 additions, alternately adding the milk in two additions.

5. Remove about $1\frac{1}{2}$ cups of the batter and place it in a small bowl. Set aside. Scrape the remaining batter into the prepared pan.

6. Fold the melted chocolate into the reserved batter. Place large spoonfuls of the chocolate batter on top of the batter in the pan. To swirl the batter, hold a table knife with the tip down. Insert the knife blade down through batter, running it gently all around the pan at least 2 times.

7. Bake 40 minutes or until the cake is golden brown and a toothpick comes out clean when inserted in the center. Let cool on a rack 10 minutes.

8. Invert the cake onto the rack and remove the pan. Turn the cake right-side up on another rack. Let cool completely. Serve immediately, or cover with an inverted bowl and store at room temperature up to 2 days.

Rum Cake

Baba au Rhum

Makes 8 to 10 servings

According to a popular story, this cake was invented by a Polish king who found his babka, a Polish yeast cake, too dry and poured a glass of rum on it. His creation was named baba, after Ali Baba of the Arabian Nights. How it became popular in Naples is not certain, but it has been for some time.

Because it is leavened with yeast rather than baking powder, baba has a spongy texture, perfect for absorbing the rum syrup. Some versions are baked in miniature muffin pans, while others have a pastry cream filling. I like to serve this with strawberries and whipped cream on the side—not typical, but delicious, and makes a lovely presentation.

1 package (2½ teaspoons) active dry yeast or instant yeast

¼ cup warm milk (100° to 110°F)

6 large eggs

2⅔ cups all-purpose flour

3 tablespoons sugar

½ teaspoon salt

¾ cup (1½ sticks) unsalted butter, at room temperature

Syrup

2 cups sugar

2 cups water

2 (2-inch) strips lemon zest

¼ cup rum

1. Grease a 10-inch tube pan.

2. Sprinkle the yeast over the warm milk. Let stand until creamy, about 1 minute, then stir until dissolved.

3. In a large mixing bowl, with an electric mixer on medium speed, beat the eggs until foamy, about 1 minute. Beat in the flour, sugar, and salt. Add the yeast and butter and beat until well blended, about 2 minutes

4. Scrape the dough into the prepared pan. Cover with plastic wrap and let stand in a warm place 1 hour or until the dough has doubled in volume.

5. Place a rack in the center of the oven. Preheat the oven to 400°F. Bake the cake 30 minutes or until it is golden and a toothpick inserted in the center comes out clean.

6. Invert the cake onto a cooling rack. Remove the pan and let cool for 10 minutes.

7. To make the syrup, combine the sugar, water, and lemon zest in a medium saucepan. Bring the mixture to a boil and stir until the sugar is dissolved, about 2 minutes. Remove the lemon zest. Stir in the rum. Set aside $^1/_4$ cup of the syrup.

8. Return the cake to the pan. With a fork, poke holes all over the surface. Slowly spoon the syrup over the cake while both are still hot. Let cool completely in the pan.

9. Just before serving, invert the cake onto a serving plate Drizzle with the remaining syrup. Serve immediately. Store covered with an overturned bowl at room temperature up to 2 days.

Grandmother's Cake

Torta della Nonna

Makes 8 servings

I couldn't decide whether to include this recipe—called torta della nonna—with the tarts or with the cakes; however, because Tuscans call it a torta, I include it with the cakes. It consists of two layers of pastry filled with a thick pastry cream. I don't know whose grandmother invented it, but everyone loves her cake. There are many variations, some including lemon flavoring.

1 cup milk

3 large egg yolks

$\frac{1}{3}$ cup sugar

1$\frac{1}{2}$ teaspoons pure vanilla extract

2 tablespoons all-purpose flour

2 tablespoons orange liqueur or rum

Dough

1$\frac{2}{3}$ cup all-purpose flour

½ cup sugar

1 teaspoon baking powder

½ teaspoon salt

½ cup (1 stick) unsalted butter, at room temperature

1 large egg, lightly beaten

1 teaspoon pure vanilla extract

1 egg yolk beaten with 1 teaspoon water, for egg wash

2 tablespoons pine nuts

Confectioner's sugar

1. In a medium saucepan, heat the milk over low heat until bubbles form around the edges. Remove from the heat.

2. In a medium bowl, whisk the egg yolks, sugar, and vanilla until pale yellow, about 5 minutes. Whisk in the flour. Gradually add the hot milk, whisking constantly. Transfer the mixture to the saucepan and cook over medium heat, stirring constantly, until boiling. Reduce the heat and simmer for 1 minute. Scrape the mixture into a bowl. Stir in the liqueur. Place a piece of plastic

wrap directly on the surface of the custard to prevent a skin from forming. Refrigerate 1 hour up to overnight.

3. Place the rack in the center of the oven. Preheat the oven to 350°F. Grease a 9 × 2–inch round cake pan.

4. Prepare the dough: In a large bowl, stir together the flour, sugar, baking powder, and salt. With a pastry blender, cut in the butter until the mixture resembles coarse crumbs. Add the egg and vanilla and stir until a dough forms. Divide the dough in half.

5. Scatter half of the dough evenly in the bottom of the prepared pan. Press the dough into the bottom of the pan and $1/2$ inch up the sides. Spread the chilled custard over the center of the dough, leaving a 1-inch border around the edge.

6. On a lightly floured surface, roll out the remaining dough to a $9^1/_2$-inch circle. Place the dough over the filling. Press the edges of the dough together to seal. Brush the egg wash over the top of the cake. Sprinkle with the pine nuts. With a small knife, make several slits in the top to allow steam to escape.

7. Bake 35 to 40 minutes, or until golden brown on top. Let cool in the pan on a rack for 10 minutes.

8. Invert the cake onto the rack, then invert onto another rack to cool completely. Sprinkle with confectioner's sugar before serving. Serve immediately, or wrap the cake in plastic wrap and refrigerate up to 8 hours. Wrap and store in the refrigerator.

Apricot Almond Cake

Torta di Albicocche e Mandorle

Makes 8 servings

Apricots and almonds are very compatible flavors. If you can't find fresh apricots, substitute peaches or nectarines.

Topping

$\frac{2}{3}$ cup sugar

$\frac{1}{4}$ cup water

12 to 14 apricots or 6 to 8 peaches, halved, pitted, and cut into $\frac{1}{4}$-inch-thick slices

Cake

1 cup all-purpose flour

1 teaspoon baking powder

$\frac{1}{2}$ teaspoon salt

$\frac{1}{2}$ cup almond paste

2 tablespoons unsalted butter

²⁄₃ cup sugar

¹⁄₂ teaspoon pure vanilla extract

2 large eggs

²⁄₃ cup milk

1. Prepare the topping: Place the sugar and water in a small heavy saucepan. Cook over medium heat, stirring occasionally, until the sugar is completely dissolved, about 3 minutes. When the mixture begins to boil, stop stirring and cook until the syrup starts to brown around the edges. Then gently swirl the pan over the heat until the syrup is an even golden brown, about 2 minutes more.

2. Protecting your hand with a pot holder, immediately pour the caramel into a 9 × 2–inch round cake pan. Tilt the pan to coat the bottom evenly. Let the caramel cool until set, about 5 minutes.

3. Place the oven rack in the center of the oven. Preheat the oven to 350°F. Arrange the sliced fruit, overlapping them slightly, in circles on top of the caramel.

4. Combine the flour, baking powder, and salt in a fine-mesh strainer set over a piece of wax paper. Sift the dry ingredients onto the paper.

5. In a large electric mixer bowl, beat the almond paste, butter, sugar, and vanilla until fluffy, about 4 minutes. Beat in the eggs one at a time, scraping the side of the bowl. Continue beating until smooth and well blended, about 4 minutes more.

6. With the mixer on low speed, stir in $1/3$ of the flour mixture. Add $1/3$ of the milk. Add the remaining flour mixture and milk in two more additions in the same way, ending with the flour. Stir just until smooth.

7. Pour the batter over the fruit. Bake 40 to 45 minutes or until the cake is golden and a toothpick inserted in the center comes out clean.

8. Let the cake cool in the pan on a wire rack 10 minutes. Run a thin metal spatula around the inside of the pan. Invert the cake onto a serving plate (the fruit will be on top) and let cool completely before serving. Serve immediately, or cover with an inverted bowl and store at room temperature up to 24 hours.

Summer Fruit Torte

Torta dell'Estate

Makes 8 servings

Soft stone fruits such as plums, apricots, peaches, and nectarines are ideal for this torte. Try making it with a combination of fruits.

12 to 16 prune plums or apricots, or 6 medium peaches or nectarines, halved, pitted, and cut into $1/2$-inch slices

1 cup all-purpose flour

1 teaspoon baking powder

$1/2$ teaspoon salt

$1/2$ cup (1 stick) unsalted butter, at room temperature

$2/3$ cup plus 2 tablespoons sugar

1 large egg

1 teaspoon grated lemon zest

1 teaspoon pure vanilla extract

Confectioner's sugar

1. Place the rack in the center of the oven. Preheat the oven to 350°F. Grease a 9-inch springform pan.

2. In a large bowl, mix together the flour, baking powder, and salt.

3. In another large bowl, beat the butter with $2/3$ cup of the sugar until light and fluffy, about 3 minutes. Beat in the egg, lemon zest, and vanilla until smooth. Add the dry ingredients and stir just until blended, about 1 minute more.

4. Scrape the batter into the prepared pan. Arrange the fruit, overlapping it slightly, on top in concentric circles. Sprinkle with the remaining 2 tablespoons of sugar.

5. Bake 45 to 50 minutes or until the cake is golden brown and a toothpick inserted in the center comes out clean.

6. Let the cake cool in the pan on a wire rack 10 minutes, then remove the rim of the pan. Let the cake cool completely. Sprinkle with confectioner's sugar before serving. Serve immediately, or cover with an overturned bowl and store at room temperature up to 24 hours.

Autumn Fruit Torte

Torta del Autunno

Makes 8 servings

Apples, pears, figs, or plums are good in this simple cake. The batter forms a top layer that does not quite cover the fruit, allowing it to peek through the surface of the cake. I like to serve it slightly warm.

1$\frac{1}{2}$ cups all-purpose flour

1 teaspoon baking powder

$\frac{1}{2}$ teaspoon salt

2 large eggs

1 cup sugar

1 teaspoon pure vanilla extract

4 tablespoons unsalted butter, melted and cooled

2 medium apples or pears, peeled, cored, and sliced into thin wedges

Confectioner's sugar

1. Place the rack in the center of the oven. Preheat the oven to 350°F. Grease and flour a 9-inch springform cake pan. Tap out the excess flour.

2. In a bowl, stir together the flour, baking powder, and salt.

3. In a large bowl, beat the eggs with the sugar and vanilla until blended, about 2 minutes. Beat in the butter. Stir in the flour mixture until just blended, about 1 minute more.

4. Spread half of the batter in the prepared pan. Cover with the fruits. Drop the remaining batter on top by spoonfuls. Spread the batter evenly over the fruits. The layer will be thin. Don't be concerned if the fruit is not completely covered.

5. Bake 30 to 35 minutes or until the cake is golden brown and a toothpick inserted in the center comes out clean.

6. Let the cake cool 10 minutes in the pan on a wire rack. Remove the rim of the pan. Cool the cake completely on the rack. Serve warm or at room temperature with a sprinkle of confectioner's sugar. Store covered with a large inverted bowl at room temperature up to 24 hours.

Polenta and Pear Cake

Dolce di Polenta

Makes 8 servings

Yellow cornmeal adds a pleasant texture and warm golden color to this rustic cake from the Veneto.

1 cup all-purpose flour

$\frac{1}{3}$ cup finely ground yellow cornmeal

1 teaspoon baking powder

$\frac{1}{2}$ teaspoon salt

$\frac{3}{4}$ cup ($1\frac{1}{2}$ sticks) unsalted butter, softened

$\frac{3}{4}$ cup plus 2 tablespoons sugar

1 teaspoon pure vanilla extract

$\frac{1}{2}$ teaspoon grated lemon zest

2 large eggs

$\frac{1}{3}$ cup milk

1 large ripe pear, cored and thinly sliced

1. Place a rack in the center of the oven. Preheat the oven to 350°F. Grease and flour a 9-inch springform pan. Tap out the excess flour.

2. In a large bowl, sift together the flour, cornmeal, baking powder, and salt.

3. In a large bowl with an electric mixer, beat the butter, gradually adding ³/₄ cup of the sugar until light and fluffy, about 3 minutes. Beat in the vanilla and lemon zest. Beat in the eggs one at time, scraping the sides of the bowl. On low speed, stir in half of the dry ingredients. Add the milk. Stir in the remaining dry ingredients just until smooth, about 1 minute.

4. Spread the batter in the prepared pan. Arrange the pear slices on top, overlapping them slightly. Sprinkle the pear with the remaining 2 tablespoons of sugar.

5. Bake 45 minutes or until the cake is golden brown and a toothpick inserted in the center comes out clean.

6. Cool the cake in the pan 10 minutes on a wire rack. Remove the pan rim and cool the cake completely on the rack. Serve immediately, or cover with a large inverted bowl and store at room temperature up to 24 hours.

Ricotta Cheesecake

Torta di Ricotta

Makes 12 servings

I like to think of this as an American-style Italian cheesecake. It is a large cake, though the flavor is delicate, with lemon zest and cinnamon. This cake is baked in a water bath so that it cooks evenly. The base of the pan is wrapped in foil to prevent the water from seeping into the pan.

1¼ cups sugar

⅓ cup all-purpose flour

½ teaspoon ground cinnamon

3 pounds whole or part-skim ricotta

8 large eggs

2 teaspoons pure vanilla extract

2 teaspoons grated lemon zest

1. Place a rack in the center of the oven. Preheat the oven to 350°F. Grease and flour a 9-inch springform pan. Tap out the excess flour. Place the pan on a 12-inch square of heavy-duty aluminum foil. Mold the foil tightly around the base and about 2 inches up the sides of the pan so that water cannot seep in.

2. In a medium bowl, stir together the sugar, flour, and cinnamon.

3. In a large mixing bowl, whisk the ricotta until smooth. Beat in the eggs, vanilla, and lemon zest until well blended. (For a smoother texture, beat the ingredients with an electric mixer or process them in a food processor.) Whisk in the dry ingredients just until blended.

4. Pour the batter into the prepared pan. Set the pan in a large roasting pan and place it in the oven. Carefully pour hot water to a depth of 1 inch in the roasting pan. Bake $1^1/_2$ hours or until the top of the cake is golden and a toothpick inserted 2 inches from the center comes out clean.

5. Turn off the oven and prop the door open slightly. Let the cake cool in the turned off oven 30 minutes. Remove the cake from the oven and remove the foil wrapping. Cool to room temperature in the pan on a wire rack.

6. Serve at room temperature or refrigerate and serve slightly chilled. Store covered with an inverted bowl in the refrigerator up to 3 days.

Sicilian Ricotta Cake

Cassata

Makes 10 to 12 servings

Cassata is the glory of Sicilian desserts. It consists of two layers of pan di Spagna (Sponge Cake) filled with sweetened, flavored ricotta. The whole cake is frosted with two icings, one of tinted almond paste and the other flavored with lemon. Sicilians decorate the cake with glistening candied fruits and almond paste cutouts so that it looks like something out of a fairy tale.

Originally served only at Easter time, cassata is now found at celebrations throughout the year.

2 Sponge Cake layers

1 pound whole or part-skim ricotta

½ cup confectioner's sugar

1 teaspoon pure vanilla extract

¼ teaspoon ground cinnamon

½ cup chopped semisweet chocolate

2 tablespoons chopped candied orange peel

Icing

4 ounces almond paste

2 or 3 drops green food coloring

2 egg whites

¼ teaspoon grated lemon zest

1 tablespoon fresh lemon juice

2 cups confectioner's sugar

Candied or dried fruits, such as cherries, pineapple, or citron

1. Prepare the sponge cake, if necessary. Then, in a large bowl with a wire whisk, beat the ricotta, sugar, vanilla, and cinnamon until smooth and creamy. Fold in the chocolate and orange peel.

2. Place one cake layer on a serving plate. Spread the ricotta mixture on top. Place the second cake layer over the filling.

3. For the decoration, crumble the almond paste into a food processor fitted with the steel blade. Add one drop of the food coloring. Process until evenly tinted a light green, adding more color if needed. Remove the almond paste and shape it into a short thick log.

4. Cut the almond paste into 4 lengthwise slices. Place one slice between two sheets of wax paper. With a rolling pin, flatten it into a narrow ribbon 3 inches long and $1/8$-inch thick. Unwrap and trim off any rough edges, reserving the scraps. Repeat with the remaining almond paste. The ribbons should be about the same width as the height of the cake. Wrap the almond paste ribbons end to end all around the sides of the cake, overlapping the ends slightly.

5. Gather the scraps of almond paste and reroll them. Cut into decorative shapes, such as stars, flowers, or leaves, with cookie cutters.

6. Prepare the icing: Whisk the egg whites, lemon zest, and juice. Add the confectioner's sugar and stir until smooth.

7. Spread the icing evenly over the top of the cake. Decorate the cake with the almond paste cutouts and the candied fruits. Cover with a large overturned bowl and refrigerate until serving time, up to 8 hours. Store leftovers covered in the refrigerator up to 2 days.

Ricotta Crumb Cake

Sbriciolata di Ricotta

Makes 8 servings

Brunch, a very American meal, is fashionable right now in Milan and other cities in northern Italy. This is my version of the ricotta-filled crumb cake I ate at brunch at a caffè not far from the Piazza del Duomo in the heart of Milan.

2½ cups all-purpose flour

½ teaspoon salt

½ teaspoon ground cinnamon

¾ cup (1½ sticks) unsalted butter

⅔ cup sugar

1 large egg

Filling

1 pound whole or part-skim ricotta

¼ cup sugar

1 teaspoon grated lemon zest

1 large egg, beaten

¼ cup raisins

Confectioner's sugar

1. Place a rack in the center of the oven. Preheat the oven to 350°F. Grease and flour a 9-inch springform pan. Tap out the excess flour.

2. In a large bowl, stir together the flour, salt, and cinnamon.

3. In a large bowl, with an electric mixer at medium speed, beat together the butter and sugar until light and fluffy, about 3 minutes. Beat in the egg. On low speed, stir in the dry ingredients until the mixture is blended and forms a firm dough, about 1 minute more.

4. Prepare the filling: Stir together the ricotta, sugar, and lemon zest until blended. Add the egg and stir well. Stir in the raisins.

5. Crumble ²/₃ of the dough into the prepared pan. Pat the crumbs firmly to form the bottom crust. Spread with the ricotta mixture, leaving a ¹/₂-inch border all around. Crumble the remaining dough over the top, scattering the crumbs evenly.

6. Bake 40 to 45 minutes or until the cake is golden brown and a toothpick inserted in the center comes out clean. Let cool in the pan on a rack 10 minutes.

7. Run a thin metal spatula around the inside of the pan. Remove the pan rim and cool the cake completely. Sprinkle with confectioner's sugar before serving. Store covered with a large inverted bowl in the refrigerator up to 2 days.

Easter Wheat-Berry Cake

La Pastiera

Wheat berries add a slightly chewy texture to this traditional Neapolitan Easter cake. This was my father's mother's recipe, which she brought with her from Procida, an island off the coast of Naples. Neapolitans love this dessert, and you will find it in bakeries and restaurants in the area all year round. Both the crust and the filling are flavored with cinnamon and orange-flower water, a delicate essence made from orange blossoms that is frequently used in southern Italian desserts. It can be found in many gourmet stores, spice shops, and ethnic markets. Substitute fresh orange juice if you cannot find it. Hulled wheat is often found in Italian markets and natural food stores, or try the mail order sources.

Dough

3 cups all-purpose flour

$1/2$ teaspoon ground cinnamon

$1/2$ teaspoon salt

$3/4$ cup ($1\frac{1}{2}$ sticks) unsalted butter, softened

1 cup confectioner's sugar

1 large egg

2 large egg yolks

2 teaspoons orange-flower water

Filling

4 ounces hulled wheat (about ½ cup)

½ teaspoon salt

½ cup (1 stick) unsalted butter, softened

1 teaspoon grated orange zest

1 pound (2 cups) whole or part-skim ricotta

4 large eggs, at room temperature

⅔ cup sugar

3 tablespoons orange-flower water

1 teaspoon ground cinnamon

½ cup very finely chopped candied citron

½ cup very finely chopped candied orange peel

Confectioner's sugar

1. Prepare the dough: In a large bowl, stir together the flour, cinnamon, and salt.

2. In a large bowl with an electric mixer on medium speed, beat the butter and confectioner's sugar until light and fluffy, about 3 minutes. Add the egg and yolks and beat until smooth. Beat in the orange-flower water. Add the dry ingredients and stir just until blended, about 1 minute more.

3. Shape $1/4$ of the dough into a disk. Make a second disk with the remaining dough. Wrap each piece in plastic wrap and chill 1 hour up to overnight.

4. Prepare the filling: Place the wheat in a large bowl, add cold water to cover, and let soak overnight in the refrigerator. Drain the wheat.

5. Place the soaked wheat in a medium saucepan with cold water to cover. Add the salt and bring to a simmer over medium heat. Cook, stirring occasionally, until the wheat is tender, 20 to 30 minutes. Drain, and place in a large bowl. Stir in the butter and orange zest. Let cool.

6. Place the rack in the lower third of the oven. Preheat the oven to 350°F. Grease and flour a 9 × 3– inch springform pan. In a large bowl, whisk together the ricotta, eggs, sugar, orange-flower water, and cinnamon. Beat until blended. Stir in the wheat mixture, citron, and candied orange peel.

7. Roll out the larger piece of dough to a 16-inch circle. Drape the dough over the rolling pin. Using the pin to lift it, fit the dough into the pan, flattening out any wrinkles against the inside of the pan. Scrape the filling onto the dough and smooth the top.

8. Roll out the smaller piece of dough to a 10-inch circle. With a fluted pastry cutter, cut the dough into $1/2$-inch-wide strips. Lay the strips across the filling in a lattice pattern. Press the ends of the strips against the dough on the sides of the pan. Trim the dough, leaving $1/2$ inch of excess all around the rim, and fold the edge of the crust over the ends of the lattice strips. Press firmly to seal.

9. Bake 1 hour 10 minutes or until the cake is golden brown on top and a toothpick inserted in the center comes out clean.

10. Let the cake cool in the pan on a rack 15 minutes. Remove the rim of the pan and let the cake cool completely on a wire rack.

Just before serving, sprinkle with confectioner's sugar. Store covered with an inverted bowl in the refrigerator up to 3 days.

Chocolate Hazelnut Cake

Torta Gianduja

Makes 8 to 10 servings

Chocolate and hazelnut, a favorite combination in Piedmont, is known as gianduja (pronounced gyan-doo-ya). You will find many candies made or filled with gianduja, gelato flavored with gianduja, and the most famous gianduja of all, Nutella, a creamy jarred chocolate hazelnut spread that Italian kids prefer to peanut butter. Gianduja is also the name of the stock character in commedia dell'arte who represents Turin, the capital city of Piedmont.

This Piedmontese cake is dark, dense, and extremely rich.

6 ounces semisweet or bittersweet chocolate

$1\frac{2}{3}$ cups hazelnuts, toasted and skinned (see How To Toast and Skin Nuts)

$\frac{1}{2}$ cup (1 stick) unsalted butter, at room temperature

1 cup sugar

5 large eggs, separated

Pinch of salt

Glaze

6 ounces semisweet or bittersweet chocolate, chopped

2 tablespoons unsalted butter

1. In the bottom half of a double boiler or in a medium saucepan, bring 2 inches of water to a simmer. Place the chocolate in the top half of the double boiler or in a bowl that will sit comfortably over the saucepan. Let the chocolate stand until softened, about 5 minutes. Stir until smooth. Let cool slightly.

2. Place the oven rack in the center of the oven. Preheat the oven to 350°F. Grease a 9 × 2–inch round cake pan.

3. In a food processor or blender, finely chop the hazelnuts. Set aside 2 tablespoons.

4. In a large bowl, with an electric mixer at medium speed, beat the butter with the sugar until light and fluffy, about 3 minutes. Add the egg yolks and beat until smooth. With a rubber spatula, stir in the chocolate and hazelnuts.

5. In a large clean bowl with clean beaters, whip the egg whites and salt on medium speed until foamy, about 1 minute. Increase the speed to high and beat until soft peaks form, about 5 minutes. With a rubber spatula, gently fold a large spoonful of the whites into the chocolate mixture to lighten it. Then gradually fold in the remainder. Scrape the batter into the prepared pan and smooth the surface. Bake 55 to 60 minutes, or until the cake is firm around the edge but slightly moist in the center.

6. Let cool in the pan for 15 minutes on a wire rack. Then unmold the cake onto a rack, invert onto another rack, and let cool completely right-side up.

7. Prepare the glaze: Bring about 2 inches of water to a simmer in the bottom half of a double boiler or a small saucepan. Place the chocolate and the butter in the top half of the double boiler or in a small heatproof bowl that fits comfortably over the saucepan. Place the bowl over the simmering water. Let stand uncovered until the chocolate is softened. Stir until smooth.

8. Place the cake on a cake rack set over a large piece of wax paper. Pour the glaze over the cake and spread it evenly over the sides and top with a long metal spatula.

9. Sprinkle the remaining 2 tablespoons of chopped nuts around the edge of the cake. Let stand in a cool place until the glaze is set.

10. Serve at room temperature. Store covered with a large inverted bowl in the refrigerator up to 3 days.

Chocolate Almond Cake

Torta Caprese

Makes 8 servings

I am not sure how this delicate cake became a specialty of Capri, but for me it is a great memento of my visits there. Serve it with whipped cream.

8 ounces semisweet or bittersweet chocolate

1 cup (2 sticks) unsalted butter, at room temperature

1 cup sugar

6 large eggs, separated, at room temperature

1½ cups almonds, very finely ground

Pinch of salt

Unsweetened cocoa powder

1. In the bottom half of a double boiler or in a medium saucepan, bring 2 inches of water to a simmer. Place the chocolate in the top half of the double boiler or in a heatproof bowl that will sit comfortably over the saucepan. Let the chocolate stand until softened, about 5 minutes. Stir until smooth. Let cool slightly.

2. Place the oven rack in the center of the oven. Preheat the oven to 350°F. Grease and flour a 9-inch round cake pan. Tap out the excess flour.

3. In a large bowl with an electric mixer at medium speed, beat the butter with $3/4$ cup of the sugar until light and fluffy, about 3 minutes. Add the egg yolks one at a time, beating well after each addition. With a rubber spatula, stir in the chocolate and the almonds.

4. In a large clean bowl with clean beaters, beat the egg whites with the salt on medium speed until foamy. Increase the speed to high and beat in the remaining $1/4$ cup of sugar. Continue to beat until the egg whites are glossy and hold soft peaks when the beaters are lifted, about 5 minutes.

5. Fold about $1/4$ of the whites into the chocolate mixture to lighten it. Gradually fold in the remaining whites.

6. Scrape the batter into the prepared pan. Bake 45 minutes or until the cake is set around the edge but soft and moist in the center and a toothpick inserted in the center comes out covered with chocolate. Let cool in the pan on a rack 10 minutes.

7. Run a thin metal spatula around the inside of the pan. Invert the cake onto a plate. Turn it right-side up onto a cooling rack. Let cool completely, then dust with cocoa powder. Serve at room temperature. Store covered with a large inverted bowl in the refrigerator up to 3 days.

Chocolate Orange Torte

Torta di Cioccolatta all' Arancia

Makes 8 servings

Chocolate and orange make an excellent combination in this unusual cake from Liguria. Be sure to use moist, flavorful candied orange peel for this cake.

6 ounces bittersweet or semisweet chocolate

6 large eggs, at room temperature, separated

²∕₃ cup sugar

2 tablespoons orange liqueur

1²∕₃ cup walnuts, toasted and very finely chopped (see How To Toast and Skin Nuts)

¹∕₃ cup finely chopped candied orange peel

Confectioner's sugar

1. Place the rack in the lower third of the oven. Preheat the oven to 350°F. Grease and flour a 9-inch springform pan, tapping out the excess flour.

2. In the bottom half of a double boiler or in a medium saucepan, bring 2 inches of water to a simmer. Place the chocolate in the top half of the double boiler or in a bowl that will sit comfortably over the saucepan. Let the chocolate stand until softened, about 5 minutes. Stir until smooth.

3. In a large bowl, with an electric mixer at medium speed, beat the egg yolks and $1/3$ cup of the sugar until thick and pale yellow, about 5 minutes. Beat in the orange liqueur. Stir in the chocolate, nuts, and orange peel.

4. In a large clean mixer bowl, beat the egg whites on medium speed until foamy. Gradually beat in the remaining $1/3$ cup of sugar. Increase the speed and beat until the whites are glossy and soft peaks form, about 5 minutes. With a rubber spatula, fold $1/3$ of the beaten whites into the chocolate mixture to lighten it. Gradually fold in the remainder.

5. Scrape the batter into the prepared pan. Bake 45 minutes or until the cake is set around the edge but still slightly moist when a toothpick is inserted in the center.

6. Cool the cake completely in the pan on a wire rack. Run a thin metal spatula around the inside of the pan to release it. Remove the rim and place the cake on a serving plate. Just before serving, sprinkle the cake with confectioner's sugar. Serve at room temperature. Store covered with a large inverted bowl in the refrigerator up to 3 days.

CPSIA information can be obtained
at www.ICGtesting.com
Printed in the USA
BVHW032257010822
643527BV00013B/314